Infectious Disease Complications of Opioid Use and Other Substance Use Disorders

Editors

SANDRA A. SPRINGER
CARLOS DEL RIO

INFECTIOUS DISEASE CLINICS OF NORTH AMERICA

www.id.theclinics.com

Consulting Editor
HELEN W. BOUCHER

September 2020 • Volume 34 • Number 3

ELSEVIER

1600 John F. Kennedy Boulevard • Suite 1800 • Philadelphia, Pennsylvania, 19103-2899.
http://www.theclinics.com

INFECTIOUS DISEASE CLINICS OF NORTH AMERICA Volume 34, Number 3
September 2020 ISSN 0891–5520, ISBN-13: 978-0-323-77785-8

Editor: Kerry Holland
Developmental Editor: Donald Mumford

Infectious Disease Clinics of North America (ISSN 0891–5520) is published in March, June, September, and December by Elsevier Inc., 360 Park Avenue South, New York, NY 10010-1710. Periodicals postage paid at New York, NY and additional mailing offices. Subscription prices are $340.00 per year for US individuals, $703.00 per year for US institutions, $100.00 per year for US students, $396.00 per year for Canadian individuals, $878.00 per year for Canadian institutions, $432.00 per year for international individuals, $878.00 per year for international institutions, $100.00 per year for Canadian students, and $200.00 per year for international students. To receive student rate, orders must be accompanied by name of affiliated institution, date of term, and the *signature* of program/residency coordinator on institution letterhead. Orders will be billed at individual rate until proof of status is received. Foreign air speed delivery is included in all *Clinics* subscription prices. All prices are subject to change without notice. **POSTMASTER**: Send address changes to *Infectious Disease Clinics of North America,* Elsevier Health Sciences Division, Subcription Customer Service, 3251 Riverport Lane, Maryland Heights, MO 63043. **Customer Service: 1-800-654-2452 (US). From outside of the US and Canada, call 1-314-447-8871. Fax: 1-314-447-8029. E-mail: JournalsCustomerService-usa@elsevier.com (print support) or JournalsOnlineSupport-usa@elsevier.com (online support).**

Infectious Disease Clinics of North America is also published in Spanish by Editorial Inter-Médica, Junin 917, 1er A 1113, Buenos Aires, Argentina.

Reprints. For copies of 100 or more, of articles in this publication, please contact the Commercial Reprints Department, Elsevier Inc., 360 Park Avenue South, New York, New York 10010-1710. Tel. 212-633-3874, Fax: 212-633-3820, E-mail: reprints@elsevier.com.

Infectious Disease Clinics of North America is covered in *MEDLINE/PubMed (Index Medicus), Current Contents/ Clinical Medicine, Science Citation Alert, SCISEARCH,* and *Research Alert.*

Contributors

CONSULTING EDITOR

HELEN W. BOUCHER, MD, FIDSA, FACP
Director, Infectious Diseases Fellowship Program, Division of Geographic Medicine and Infectious Diseases, Tufts Medical Center, Associate Professor of Medicine, Tufts University School of Medicine, Boston, Massachusetts

EDITORS

SANDRA A. SPRINGER, MD
Associate Professor of Medicine, Department of Internal Medicine, Section of Infectious Diseases, Yale School of Medicine, Center for Interdisciplinary Research on AIDS, Yale School of Public Health, New Haven, Connecticut; Veterans Affairs Connecticut Healthcare System, West Haven, Connecticut

CARLOS DEL RIO, MD
Distinguished Professor of Medicine, Division of Infectious Diseases, Executive Associate Dean, Emory School of Medicine, Professor of Global Health and Epidemiology, Rollins School of Public Health, Emory University, Atlanta, Georgia

AUTHORS

WOLLELAW AGMAS, MD
Infectious Disease Fellow, Maine Medical Center/Tufts University School of Medicine, Portland, Maine

JOSHUA A. BAROCAS, MD
Assistant Professor of Medicine, Section of Infectious Diseases, Boston Medical Center, Boston University School of Medicine, Boston, Massachusetts

HEATHER M. BRADLEY, PhD
Department of Epidemiology, School of Public Health, Georgia State University, Atlanta, Georgia

EVELYN VILLACORTA CARI, MD
Fellow, Division of Infectious Disease, University of Kentucky College of Medicine, Lexington, Kentucky

TERESA A. CHUENG, MD, MPH
Division of Infectious Diseases, Department of Medicine, University of Miami Miller School of Medicine, Jackson Memorial Hospital, Jackson Health System, Miami, Florida

JONATHAN A. COLASANTI, MD, MSPH
Assistant Professor, Department of Medicine, Division of Infectious Diseases, Emory University, Atlanta, Georgia

ELLEN F. EATON, MD, MSPH
Assistant Professor of Medicine, Division of Infectious Disease, The University of Alabama at Birmingham, Birmingham, Alabama

AARON FOX, MD
Associate Professor of Medicine, Department of Internal Medicine, Montefiore Medical Center, Bronx, New York

ALYSSA GRIMSHAW, MSLIS
Harvey Cushing/John Hay Whitney Medical Library, Yale University, New Haven, Connecticut

CRAIG G. GUNDERSON, MD
Department of Internal Medicine, Section of General Internal Medicine, Yale School of Medicine, New Haven, Connecticut; Veterans Affairs Connecticut Healthcare System, West Haven, Connecticut

HERMIONE HURLEY, MBChB, BE
Assistant Professor, Center for Addiction Medicine, Denver Health and Hospital Authority, Denver, Colorado

TIMOTHY JENKINS, MD, MSc
Associate Professor, Division of Infectious Disease, Denver Health and Hospital Authority, Denver, Colorado

SIMEON D. KIMMEL, MD, MA
Assistant Professor of Medicine, Sections of Infectious Diseases and General Internal Medicine, Department of Medicine, Boston Medical Center, Boston University School of Medicine, Boston, Massachusetts

NANCY S. MILLER, MD
Associate Professor, Department of Pathology and Laboratory Medicine, Boston Medical Center, Boston University School of Medicine, Boston, Massachusetts

KATHERINE NENNINGER, MD
Preventive Medicine, Clinical Instructor in Medicine, Maine Medical Center/Tufts University School of Medicine, Portland, Maine

ANK NIJHAWAN, MD, MPH, MSCS
Associate Professor of Internal Medicine, Division of Infectious Diseases, Department of Internal Medicine, The University of Texas Southwestern Medical Center, Dallas, Texas

JOSIAH D. RICH, MD, MPH
Professor of Medicine and Epidemiology, Departments of Medicine and Epidemiology, Brown University, Providence, Rhode Island

CARLOS DEL RIO, MD
Distinguished Professor of Medicine, Division of Infectious Diseases, Executive Associate Dean, Emory School of Medicine, Professor of Global Health and Epidemiology, Rollins School of Public Health, Emory University, Atlanta, Georgia

ELI S. ROSENBERG, PhD
Department of Epidemiology and Biostatistics, School of Public Health, University at Albany, State University of New York, Albany, New York; Epidemiology, Emory University Rollins School of Public Health, Atlanta, Georgia

CARLOS S. SALDANA, MD
Division of Infectious Diseases, Emory School of Medicine, Atlanta, Georgia

JEFFREY H. SAMET, MD, MA, MPH
The John Noble Professor of General Internal Medicine, Clinical Addiction Research and Education Unit, Section of General Internal Medicine, Department of Medicine, Boston University School of Medicine, Boston Medical Center, Department of Community Health Sciences, Boston University School of Public Health, Boston, Massachusetts

MARCOS C. SCHECHTER, MD
Division of Infectious Diseases, Department of Medicine, Emory University, Atlanta, Georgia

ASHER SCHRANZ, MD, MPH
Assistant Professor of Medicine, Division of Infectious Diseases, The University of North Carolina at Chapel Hill, Chapel Hill, North Carolina

DAVID P. SEROTA, MD, MSc
Division of Infectious Diseases, Department of Medicine, University of Miami Miller School of Medicine, Miami, Florida

NIKHIL SEVAL, MD
Department of Internal Medicine, Section of Infectious Diseases, Yale School of Medicine, New Haven, Connecticut

MONICA SIKKA, MD
Assistant Professor, Division of Infectious Diseases, Oregon Health & Science University, Portland, Oregon

SANDRA A. SPRINGER, MD
Associate Professor of Medicine, Department of Internal Medicine, Section of Infectious Diseases, Yale School of Medicine, Center for Interdisciplinary Research on AIDS, Yale School of Public Health, New Haven, Connecticut; Veterans Affairs Connecticut Healthcare System, West Haven, Connecticut

PATRICK SEAN SULLIVAN, DVM, PhD
Professor, Department of Epidemiology, Rollins School of Public Health, Emory University, Atlanta, Georgia

KINNA THAKARAR, DO, MPH
Infectious Disease and Addiction Medicine, Assistant Professor of Medicine, Maine Medical Center/Tufts University School of Medicine, South Portland, Maine

ALICE THORNTON, MD
Professor of Medicine, Chief, Division of Infectious Disease, University of Kentucky College of Medicine, Lexington, Kentucky

THERESA VETTESE, MD
Associate Professor, Department of Medicine, Division of General Internal Medicine and Geriatrics, Emory University, Emory School of Medicine, Atlanta, Georgia

DARSHALI A. VYAS, MD
Department of Medicine, Massachusetts General Hospital, Boston, Massachusetts

DANIEL WINETSKY, MD, MS
Postdoctoral Fellow, Division of Infectious Diseases, Department of Internal Medicine, Columbia University Irving Medical Center, HIV Center for Clinical and Behavioral Studies at Columbia University and New York State Psychiatric Institute, New York, New York

ALYSSE G. WURCEL, MD, MS
Department of Medicine, Division of Geographic Medicine and Infectious Diseases, Tufts University School of Medicine, Tufts Medical Center, Boston, Massachusetts

Contents

> Opioid use disorder is complex and not easily quantified among US populations because there are no dedicated reporting systems in place. We review indicators of opioid use disorder available at the state and county (human immunodeficiency virus [HIV] diagnoses among people who inject drugs, hepatitis C diagnosis in people <50 years, opioid overdose death rates, and opioid prescription rate). The interpretation of the ecological results and the visualization of indicators at the local level will provide actionable insights for clinicians and public health officials seeking to mitigate the consequences of opioid use disorder at the patient and community levels.

> Increased infections from injection drug use harm patients and are costly to the health care system. The impact on clinical microbiology laboratories is less recognized. Microbiology laboratories face increased test volume and test complexity from the spectrum and burden of pathogens associated with injection drug use, which lead to diagnostic challenges and overtaxed resources. We describe stressed workflows, pathogens that defy protocols, and limits of current technologies. Laboratories may benefit from protocol revisions, additional resources, workflow oversight, and improved communication with clinical providers to optimally meet challenges associated with this public health crisis.

> Infective endocarditis associated with injection drug use (IDU-IE) is markedly increasing in the United States and Canada. Long-term outcomes are dismal and stem from insufficient substance use disorder treatment. In this review, we summarize the principles of antimicrobial and surgical management for infective endocarditis associated with injection drug use. We discuss approaches to opioid use disorder care and harm reduction in the inpatient setting and review opportunities to address preventable infections among persons injecting drugs. We highlight barriers to implementing optimal treatment and consider novel approaches that may reshape infective endocarditis associated with injection drug use treatment in coming years.

INFECTIOUS DISEASE CLINICS OF NORTH AMERICA

THE CLINICS ARE AVAILABLE ONLINE!
Access your subscription at:
www.theclinics.com

Preface

Addressing the Intersection of Infectious Disease Epidemics and Opioid and Substance Use Epidemics

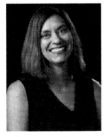 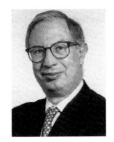

Sandra A. Springer, MD   Carlos del Rio, MD
Editors

The current opioid use disorder (OUD) and nonopioid substance use epidemics in the United States have resulted in an increase in infections among persons who use drugs (PWUD), magnifying the morbidity and mortality associated with illicit substance use. Such infections that are increasing related to illicit opioid and other drug use include hepatitis C virus (HCV), hepatitis B virus, human immunodeficiency virus (HIV), invasive bacterial and fungal infections (including *Staphylococcus aureus* bacteremia, fungemia, endocarditis, skin and soft tissue infections), and bone and joint infections, among others. Illicitly manufactured fentanyl or heroin combined with stimulants like cocaine and methamphetamine has led to new HIV outbreaks among PWUD throughout the country as well as increased overdose deaths. Persons with co-occurring drug use–related infections represent some of the most severely ill patients. Integrating treatment for the underlying substance use disorder with the associated infectious disease is an important opportunity to intervene, both to improve patients' outcomes and to reduce the public health risk of infectious disease transmission.

In this special issue of *Infectious Disease Clinics of North America* that is devoted to Infectious Complications of Opioid Use and Other Substance Use Disorders, specific articles discuss the impact substance use, and specifically, opioid use has had on individual infectious diseases like HIV, HCV, endocarditis, skin and soft tissue infections, and bone and joint infections, as well as the management of these infections with the substance use disorders within the hospital, the community, and the criminal justice settings. Furthermore, this issue includes specific articles on the geography of infectious disease related to the opioid epidemic. The special issue is strengthened by

Infect Dis Clin N Am 34 (2020) xiii–xiv
https://doi.org/10.1016/j.idc.2020.06.016
0891-5520/20/© 2020 Published by Elsevier Inc.

including specific articles addressing the microbiology and algorithms to diagnose infections related to substance use as well as specific potential novel antimicrobial treatments to consider using for those with infectious diseases related to substance use. Importantly, this special issue also addresses harm reduction services like syringe service programs on the impact of reducing infectious disease complications of opioid and other substance use as well as the management of pain in persons with co-occurring opioid and other substance use disorders in the setting of associated infectious disease complications. Last, a commentary focuses on the lessons learned from earlier responses to the HIV epidemic in the United States that could be used to combat the current opioid and other substance use epidemics that are fueling new HIV and other infectious disease epidemics. Since the time the articles in this special issue were written and accepted in January of 2019 the COVID-19 pandemic has changed the world and considerations of integration of treatments of both infectious diseases and opioid use disorder prevention and treatments are even more urgent.

Sandra A. Springer, MD
Department of Internal Medicine
Section of Infectious Disease
Yale AIDS Program
135 College Street, Suite 323
New Haven, CT 06510, USA

Carlos del Rio, MD
Department of Medicine
Division of Infectious Diseases
Emory University School of Medicine
69 Jesse Hill Jr. Drive
Faculty Office Building, Room 201
Atlanta, GA 30303, USA

E-mail addresses:
sandra.springer@yale.edu (S.A. Springer)
cdelrio@emory.edu (C. del Rio)

The Geography of Opioid Use Disorder
A Data Triangulation Approach

Patrick Sean Sullivan, DVM, PhD*, Heather M. Bradley, PhD,
Carlos del Rio, MD, Eli S. Rosenberg, PhD

KEYWORDS

- Opioid use epidemic • Opioid use disorder • Indicators • Data triangulation
- HIV diagnosis in PWID • HCV diagnosis • Opioid overdose death rate
- Opioid prescription rate

KEY POINTS

- The opioid use epidemic in the US is an important driver of HIV and HCV infections, but there no direct data sources to identify problematic opioid use.
- Several data sources, including HIV diagnoses, HCV diagnoses in younger people, opioid prescription rate and opioid overdose death rate, have different strengths and weaknesses as indicators of opioid use disorder.
- Because informative data systems have different strengths and weaknesses, a data triangulation approach is needed to identify patterns of opioid use disorder and recommend programmatic responses.

INTRODUCTION

The opioid use epidemic in the United States came into broad public view during a localized outbreak of human immunodeficiency virus (HIV) infection in southern Indiana in 2015.[1] By the time of that outbreak, the rate of drug poisoning deaths had nearly tripled since 2000, with most of that increase attributed to opioid-related deaths,[2] and 1.9 million American adults met criteria for a prescription opioid use disorder (OUD).[3] The outbreak in Scott County brought attention to a national problem through the lens of a specific community. However, the geography of problematic opioid use is much broader than rural midwestern communities, and follows a very different geographic pattern of impact compared with many chronic (eg, diabetes, hypertension, obesity) or infectious diseases (HIV, sexually transmitted infections); both chronic and infectious diseases have

This work was supported by the following NIH grants: P30AI050409, R01DA045612, R01DA038196, DA051302.
Epidemiology, Emory University Rollins School of Public Health, 1518 Clifton Road Northeast, Atlanta, GA 30322, USA
* Corresponding author.
E-mail address: pssulli@emory.edu

disproportionate impact in the South and major urban areas throughout the country. The geographic distribution of OUD speaks to underlying characteristics of opioid users and settings of opioid use, and, most importantly, to the need for interventions in parts of the United States that are often underserved by preventive health services.

There are a variety of indicators that can be used to understand the geography of OUD. In the past, data from existing surveillance systems for infectious diseases that can be transmitted by needle sharing have been used to identify trends in injection drug use (IDU). For example, trends in HIV diagnoses related to IDU and hepatitis C virus (HCV) diagnoses (especially in younger people) have been used to provide context to evolving opioid epidemics.[4] Relying on existing infectious disease surveillance systems is cost efficient, but HIV and HCV diagnoses are not specific to OUD. HIV is also relatively insensitive as an indicator of IDU because the efficiency of transmission of HIV is less than for HCV.[4] Other proxies for IDU behaviors, including skin infections and infectious endocarditis, also lack specificity for opioid injection, may be transient, and are not reportable conditions. Infectious endocarditis is an especially important indicator of OUD, because it is the most serious infectious consequence of IDU but is not monitored in any systematic way. The Drug Abuse Warning Network Emergency Department data system collects data on drug-related emergency department visits but focuses only on drugs related to the reason for the medical visit, which decreases the sensitivity of this system for understanding the scope of OUD.[5] Cause of death data from the National Vital Statistics System can provide high-quality data about specific drug use, but may be variable in quality because the patterns of testing for specific drugs in overdose cases vary by coroner or medical examiner jurisdiction and budgetary constraints associated with drug testing.[6]

Here, we review 4 indicators in terms of contributions toward our understanding of geographic patterns and temporal trends in OUD: percent of new HIV diagnoses attributable to IDU, HCV infections, the opioid prescription rate, and opioid-related overdose death rate. We discuss what is currently known about how each indicator varies geographically, at which level of geographic granularity the indicator can be meaningfully analyzed, and potential biases arising from use of each indicator as a signal for geographic patterns and temporal trends in the opioid epidemic. We conclude with a summary of geographic patterns from all 4 indicators and discussion of additional data needs.

DATA SOURCES

New Human Immunodeficiency Virus Diagnoses Attributable to Intravenous Drug Use

For number of HIV diagnoses attributed to IDU and proportions of HIV diagnoses among people who inject drugs (PWID) by state, we used data from the National Center for HIV/AIDS, Viral Hepatitis, STD, and TB Prevention Atlas and from AIDSVu.org. New diagnoses of HIV infection are reportable by law in all US jurisdictions to state/territorial health departments, who submit name-based diagnoses to the Centers for Disease Control and Prevention (CDC),[7] which deduplicates this information and makes summaries available on public repositories such as the National Center for HIV/AIDS, Viral Hepatitis, STD, and TB Prevention Atlas+[8] and AIDSVu.org[9] HIV diagnostic data are typically presented as 1-year totals, with a less than 2-year lag in national reporting[10] and often more timely data availability at the state level.[11]

Hepatitis C Virus Infections Among Persons Less than 50 Years of Age

For estimated numbers of people living with HCV we used a combination of National Health and Nutrition Examination Survey (NHANES) data and census data to produce population-based estimates, as previously described.[12–14] Briefly, NHANES estimates for HCV viral detection were used to calculate direct weighted estimates of national hepatitis C prevalence. The 2012 to 2016 American Community Survey microdata samples were used to generate estimated population totals within each state, stratified by sex, race/ethnicity, and birth cohort. These state-by-strata population totals were multiplied by the stratified Hepatitis C prevalence estimates to generate crude state-level estimates. National Vital Statistics System mortality data and intercensal population totals were used to model the HCV-related and narcotic overdose death rates in the same strata by state.

Within strata, these 2 mortality rates were combined using weights computed from data-driven assumptions about the proportion of HCV prevalence in a given birth cohort that was likely to be attributable to IDU. The combined mortality rates were multiplied by state-by-strata prevalence estimates to generate mortality-adjusted HCV prevalence totals in each stratum in each state. These totals were summed within states across strata, and the numbers of additional prevalent HCV infections estimated from populations unsampled by NHANES were added to state-specific estimates. For the stratified estimates, state- and strata-specific hepatitis C prevalence among populations unsampled by NHANES were estimated in a way that reflected state- and strata-specific hepatitis C estimates derived from NHANES.

Opioid Prescription Rates

Data on opioid prescription rates per population size are publicly available through https://www.cdc.gov/drugoverdose/ and are sourced from the IQVIA Transactional Data Warehouse (Durham, NC). IQVIA data are collected from a sample of approximately 50,000 retail pharmacies that together dispense 90% of retail prescriptions nationally. Prescriptions are recorded regardless of initial or refill status and payment type. Opioid prescriptions, include buprenorphine, codeine, fentanyl, hydrocodone, hydromorphone, methadone, morphine, oxycodone, oxymorphone, propoxyphene, tapentadol, and tramadol. US Census data were used for population size denominators.

Opioid-Related Overdose Death Rate

Data for opioid-related deaths were obtained from CDC WONDER, using *International Classification of Diseases, 10th Revision* codes consistent with CDC reporting of drug overdose deaths (eg, X40-X44, X60-X64, X85, and Y10-Y14)[15] with T-codes indicative of an opioid-related cause (eg, T40.1-T40.4, T40.6).[2,16]

INDICATORS
New Human Immunodeficiency Virus Infection Diagnoses Attributable to Intravenous Drug Use

In most states, 7% or fewer of HIV diagnoses were attributable to IDU in 2017 (**Fig. 1**). States with higher proportions of HIV infections attributed to IDU were concentrated in central Appalachia and the Northeast. Many of the states with large proportions of HIV infections attributable to IDU are also states with overall low HIV prevalence. West Virginia, Kentucky, New Hampshire, Vermont, and Maine all had less than 200 persons/ 100,000 population living with HIV in 2016,[9] yet at least 10% of new infections were attributed to IDU.

The high levels of risk factor completeness for HIV cases render HIV infections attributed to IDUs a highly sensitive signal of individuals' IDU history. Yet the long latency of HIV infection, in conjunction with infrequent testing for PWID,[17,18] may render this less specific in terms of the timing of infection and may in turn result in geographic

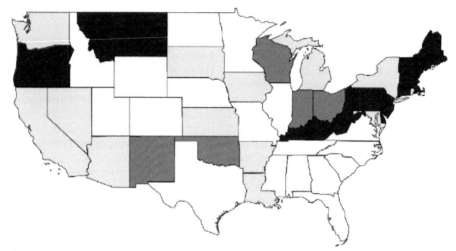

Fig. 1. Percent of HIV diagnoses attributed to IDU, by US state, 2017.

misclassification, because a persons' residence at diagnosis may be discordant from that at the time of infection. These concerns about geographic misclassification are heightened when considering using persons living with an HIV diagnosis as an indicator for OUD, because HIV is a lifelong, chronic infection.

Although data on new HIV diagnoses overall are publicly available in most states at the county level, new diagnoses attributable to IDU are available at the state level (AIDSVu), although some states and cities individually release these data at finer levels. This lack of geographic resolution is in part owing to HIV infection being a relatively rare consequence of IDU, primarily owing to the low per act acquisition risk associated with injection,[19] compared with other bloodborne viruses such as hepatitis B or C.[4]

Thus, given the rareness of a new IDU HIV diagnoses, this indicator functionally may be suppressed or not very informative given the sparseness of the information. HIV diagnoses in a specific subgroup are suppressed for groups with 1 to 4 cases in a year in a specific geographic unit, resulting in missingness either because areas have small populations (even if infection rates are higher), or in areas that have strong prevention programs. For example, data in Indiana and New York City are both sparsely reported, despite very different epidemic situations. Indiana is more sparsely populated with IDU and has a higher rate of new infections in IDU, and New York City has a higher population of IDU with lower acquisition rates. In contrast, this sparseness is amenable to the detection of HIV transmission clusters and outbreaks (eg, in West Virginia,[20] Indiana,[1] and less urban parts of Massachusetts[21]).

There is the potential for bias in eliciting IDU as a risk factor. The setting for the test (community-based organization, physician, laboratory), provider comfort/ability in eliciting risk factors, and a patient's comfort in disclosing risk may lead toward undercounting of IDU as a risk factor.[22] Some of these biases may be differential by urbanicity given variations in provider types, training, and the landscape of stigma toward PWID.[23–25]

Hepatitis C Virus Prevalence Among Persons Less than 50 Years of Age

HCV surveillance data quality differs across state and local jurisdictions, and standardized estimates of HCV infection by state are only available through modeling approaches (**Fig. 2**).[12–14] Here, we present prevalent HCV infections among persons aged less than 50 years of age by state as previously published modeled estimates[12] and as described in data sources. Estimated rates of HCV infection among persons aged less than 50 years of age were concentrated in central Appalachia (Pennsylvania, Ohio, Kentucky, West Virginia, and Tennessee), and West Virginia had the highest rate of infection among this age group in the country. This indicator is limited to persons aged less than 50, because these infections are more likely to be associated with IDU compared with infections among Baby Boomers (born between 1945 and 1965). HCV infections among Baby Boomers were generally acquired in the distant past via blood products or previous IDU. Among an estimated 44,700 acute HCV infections in 2017, most were among those less than 40 years of age and associated with IDU.[26]

Given the higher per act risk for HCV, compared with HIV, HCV infections are in theory a more sensitive and abundant signal for tracking IDU epidemics. HCV has a higher per act transmission rate per episode of needle sharing (250/10,000 acts)[27,28] than does HIV (63/10,000 acts).[19] Relatedly, HCV infections are often a leading and more prevalent indicator for subsequent HIV infections in outbreak settings.[29,30] The use of HCV diagnoses in younger people as markers for underlying HCV incidence in the population is complicated by factors that include the ability for at least one-quarter of infected persons to spontaneously clear infection, a multidecade latency period of chronic infection, and possibly lower awareness and screening rates among PWID.[31]

Another challenge for using HCV infections an indicator of OUD and associated IDU behavior is inconsistencies in how diagnoses are reported to states and to CDC. HCV diagnoses are submitted to local health departments and reported to CDC under 2 case definitions, one for its acute phase and the other for chronic phase, via the National Notifiable Diseases Surveillance System. As of 2017, 44 states reported acute

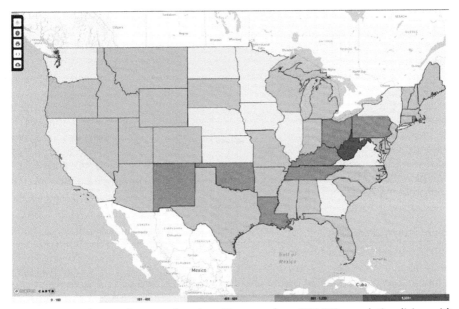

Fig. 2. Estimated rate of persons less than 50 years of age/100,000 population living with hepatitis C, by state, United States, 2013 to 2016.

HCV cases and 39 reported chronic HCV cases to CDC, with the remainder not including HCV as a legally reportable condition or not submitting data to CDC. Unlike for HIV, submissions to CDC are not name-based, precluding deduplication across jurisdictions and national-level mortality matching. Because of stringent criteria and low levels of diagnosis during the acute phase, only about 3000 acute cases are reported by CDC annually and most new diagnoses reported are chronic (143,286 in 2017). These differences in reporting across jurisdiction make geographic comparisons of HCV infections using surveillance data difficult.

Because of the heterogeneity in state submissions to the CDC, stringent case criteria, and limited stratifications available nationally, individual state-level reports often offer more detail into local HCV trends that might inform the OUD epidemic. These data come with the drawback of less standardization of how case definitions are operationalized and reporting formats between jurisdictions. Complicating this all substantially is that, relative to HIV, fewer federal resources are made available to jurisdictions for HCV surveillance, resulting in lower levels of data quality, in terms of complete reporting, completeness of demographic and risk factors, case investigations. For example, among 2017 acute diagnoses reported CDC, 48% were missing risk factor data.

Acute HCV infections overall, among those less than 50 years, and among those with reported IDU risk factors are all useful indicators for understanding trends in new IDU-associated infections. The total acute infections is available from the CDC at the state level, whereas age and IDU risk factor estimates are provided only for the national total. Given the low levels of acute infections reported to the CDC relative to chronic cases, trends in reported chronic cases among persons less than 50 years of age is another marker for IDU-associated transmission, but these data are not summarized by the CDC at any level of geography.

Both HIV and HCV diagnoses attributable to IDU have a strong correlation to OUD, because many PWID are a subset of those with OUD. Yet there are several key sources of potential sources of misalignment. First, harm reduction activities like syringe exchange lower HCV/HIV acquisition risk, but do not directly address addiction. Thus, in places with legal and more widespread access to syringe exchange,[32] one would expect greater discordance between HIV/HCV risk and OUD, controlling for drug treatment access. Conversely, in places with fewer harm reduction resources (eg, parts of Appalachia and the South), one expects tighter relationship between HIV/HCV risk and OUD. Additionally, HIV/HCV risk attributable to IDU is partly independent of the specific substance being injected, other than the pathways by which specific substances may influence injection frequency and other risk behaviors.[33] The makeup of the drug supply varies geographically and by urbanicity. Stimulant use and injection, notably methamphetamine, is increasing in a number of states and these nonopioid substances may accordingly disproportionately influence HCV/HIV risk in those places.[34] This information is likely to induce meaningful geographic variation in the relationship between HCV/HIV diagnoses and underlying prevalence of persons with OUD.

Opioid Prescription Rate

In 2017, the rate of opioid prescriptions per 100 population were generally highest in the Southeast and central Appalachia (**Fig. 3**). Nearly one-quarter of states had prescription rates higher than 74 opioid prescriptions dispensed per 100 persons during 2017. The opioid prescription rate has declined nationally since 2012, from a high of 81 of 100 persons in 2012 to 59 of 100 in 2017, but this decrease has been differential by geography.[35,36]

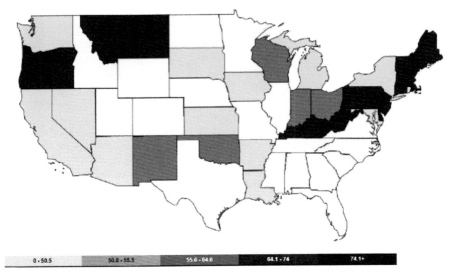

Fig. 3. Opioid prescription rate per 100,000 population by state, 2017.

Opioid prescription data are publicly available at both the state and county levels, currently from 2006 to 2017. Completeness of data is high and has improved over time, and the percentage of counties with available data increased from 88% in 2006 to 94% in 2017. Opioid prescription data are robust, relatively timely, and are collected from a sample of pharmacies representing most prescriptions dispensed in the United States. However, the opioid prescription rate was likely a more informative geographic indicator of OUD before 2010, when most drug overdose deaths were attributable to more commonly prescribed opioids versus rarely prescribed synthetic opioids, such as fentanyl, or illicit opioids such as heroin.[37–39] As the percentage of drug overdose deaths attributable to nonprescription opioids has increased, opioid prescription rate may be a less specific signal of OUD, which is increasingly associated with illicit, nonprescription opioids.

OUD attributable to prescription opioids is also somewhat undercaptured by this indicator owing to prescription opioids that are obtained illegally and outside the pharmacy setting. It is not possible to measure how much illegal sales of prescription opioids decrease the sensitivity of this indicator, but highly likely that this issue with sensitivity varies geographically. Additionally, the extent to which prescription versus nonprescription opioids are responsible for OUD prevalence varies considerably by geography,[37] further complicating geographic comparisons. The specificity of opioid prescription rate for signaling OUD is compromised by legitimate use of prescription opioids for pain management, and it is difficult to know to what extent this issue may affect geographic comparisons.

Opioid-Related Overdose Death Rate

In 2018, the highest state-specific opioid overdose death rate was reported in West Virginia (38.2/100,000) (**Fig. 4**). By region, higher opioid overdose death rates were reported in Appalachia and the Northeastern United States; of the top 10 death rates by state, 7 were in the Northeast and 4 were Appalachian states (Pennsylvania is included in both groups). Of the lowest 10 opioid overdose death rates by state, 5 were in the Midwest, 3 were in the West, and 2 were in the South.

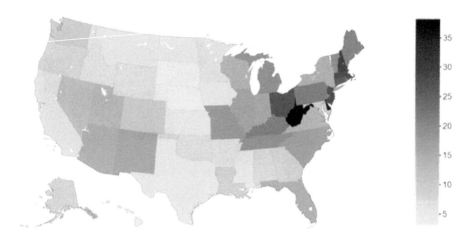

Fig. 4. Death rate attributable to opioid overdose per 100,000 population by state, United States, 2018.

The opioid-related overdose death rate is available at both state and county levels by year through CDC WONDER, which includes multiple cause of death data by cause and decedent characteristics.[40] This indicator can be used to assess geographic patterns and trends down to the county level. Importantly, opioid-related overdose deaths can be further stratified by those attributed to prescription, synthetic, and illicit opioids.[41]

Opioid-related drug overdose is a highly specific indicator of OUD. Deaths in the United States are robustly recorded in vital records, and those indicating opioid-related overdose are based on toxicology screening on autopsy and are likely to be true representations of OUD. Specificity is diminished, however, when multiple drugs are detected on toxicology, making it unclear how to attribute an overdose death.[42] This indicator may have suboptimal sensitivity for signaling geographic patterns and trends in OUD, however, owing to both geographic variability in both completeness of recording drug-specific overdose deaths and resources invested in overdose prevention among persons with OUD.

Drug overdose deaths are ascertained using a multistep process with several opportunities for misclassification. Physicians, coroners, or medical examiners record multiple causes of deaths on death certificates, and these causes of death are classified using standardized algorithms by CDC using the *International Classification of Diseases, 10th Revision*, cause of death and toxicology codes. However, when postmortem toxicology testing does not occur, T-codes will not be recorded, and drug overdose deaths will not be classified according to a specific drug type. This happens disproportionally in settings with limited death investigation resources or non-standardized toxicology testing procedures, complicating geographic comparisons.[43,44] The completeness of T-codes has increased over time as resources invested in monitoring drug overdose deaths has increased,[45] but a disparity in completeness remains in urban versus rural areas and in areas with medical examiners versus coroners, which are disproportionately rural.[43]

Geographic variability in overdose prevention interventions also compromises the sensitivity of opioid overdose deaths for signaling geographic patterns in OUD. Harm reduction strategies such as community-level distribution of naloxone, provision of test strips for the detection of contaminated drugs, and polices such as Good

Samaritan laws may all prevent overdose deaths among persons with OUD.[46–48] These interventions and policies are supported and implemented differently by geography,[49] however, and the lack of standardized data on availability of overdose death prevention interventions by geography is a limitation of using this indicator to monitor geographic patterns in OUD.

DISCUSSION

The different types of opioid data available by geography show some commonalities and some distinctions. For example, Appalachian states are disproportionately heavily impacted in all indicators, but Tennessee is in the lowest quartile of HIV diagnoses. Such discrepancies might result from other prevention modalities that would mitigate HIV transmission, but not HCV transmission or overdose deaths, such as lower prevalence of unsuppressed HIV viral load levels in PWID. Similarly, some Northeastern states like Massachusetts, Vermont, and New Hampshire have high levels of HIV diagnoses among PWID, but relatively low opioid prescription rates. In the West, Oregon, Idaho, and Montana stand out as states that in the upper quartiles of multiple indicators; these consistent patterns of indicators suggest concerns across dimensions of opioid prescriptions, overdose, and associated infectious diseases. In such areas, there are opportunities both to address the prevalence of OUD, and to broadly implement harm reduction programs (such as syringe exchange) to decrease opioid misuse and to decrease the infectious consequences of needle sharing. We recognize that such interpretations of state across indicators are subject to ecological fallacy, in that we do not know that those prescribed opioids, acquiring HCV and HIV and dying from opioid overdose are the same people.[50]

Despite these limitations, ecological comparisons across indicators by geography provide signals about where the OUD epidemic is concentrated and where it is heading. Ultimately, data at finer geographic resolutions are needed to better understand individual and community risk factors for OUD and to inform local resource allocation and intervention implementation. For example, supplemental surveillance systems such as the National HIV Behavioral System[17,51,52] and the Medical Monitoring Project[53] use targeted sampling and individual interviews to routinely assess risk factors among persons with HIV risk and health status and behaviors among persons living with HIV. These data are collected by states and cities and allow jurisdictions to understand local patterns while also allowing data to be pooled for national estimates. Similarly, the STD [sexually transmitted disease] Surveillance Network collects geographically-specific data from sexually transmitted disease clinics and individuals diagnosed with gonorrhea to provide enhanced data on demographic characteristics, risk behaviors, and unmet needs for care among persons diagnosed with gonorrhea.[54,55]

Supplemental surveillance systems such as these provide a depth of information at the person level that is not available from core HIV and sexually transmitted disease case reporting. Prevalent OUD may be less likely to be diagnosed than either HIV or gonorrhea and is not a reportable condition, complicating sampling for possible supplemental surveillance systems for OUD, and creative solutions are needed to collect routine information from persons with high OUD risk. Data from currently on-going networks of research studies such as those funded by National Institute of Health's Helping to End Addiction Long-term (HEAL) Initiative,[56] will also be helpful for understanding geographic patterns in OUD. Standardized data collection systems and a centralized repository for research data, particularly for multisite research projects, could make information for geographic comparisons more readily accessible.

In addition to geography, characteristics of place are also important considerations for understanding patterns in the OUD epidemic. Social determinants of health such as per capita income, workforce characteristics, and urbanicity are associated with both OUD risk and prevention and treatment outcomes when measured at the county level.[29,57–59] An emerging literature[58–60] suggests that these kinds of population characteristics cluster by geography and can help to identify places with high OUD risk. Findings suggest, for example, that areas with large proportions of the population involved in the mining industry, with high levels of unemployment, or with high incarceration rates have a higher risk for opioid-related overdose deaths. Particularly When these characteristics are observed in nonurban areas, they are also associated with less availability of OUD treatment services.[60] This literature indicates that structural factors interact with opioid availability to determine the trajectory of the OUD epidemic in a particular place.[29,61] Research elucidating factors underlying geographic differences in OUD prevalence provides context for understanding OUD risk, and provides critical information for resource allocation and tailoring prevention and treatment interventions.

The CDC has recently implemented several novel surveillance systems to address drug overdose that, as they mature, will provide important new insights about opioid and other drug epidemics.[62] Enhanced State Opioid Overdose Surveillance (ESOOS) funding provides support for states to collect more timely and complete data on both fatal and nonfatal overdose. ESOOS was launched in 12 states in 2016 and expanded since that time to include 47 states. A major focus of ESOOS is increasing the use of syndromic data from emergency rooms and emergency medical services for a better understanding of the number and characteristics of nonfatal overdoses. ESOOS-funded states also conduct extensive death scene investigations for overdose deaths and report information on toxicology, route of drug administration, and other pertinent information about decedents to the State Unintentional Drug Overdose Reporting System. These data sources are likely to provide more drug-specific information about both nonfatal and fatal overdoses than was previously available through the National Vital Statistics System and CDC WONDER.

Understanding the geography of OUD is important at the state and local levels to identify failures of prevention and to construct a public health program that addresses the specific needs indicated by the aggregate indicators for the jurisdiction. For example, many Appalachian states likely need a range of public health interventions, including interventions with providers to reduce decrease opioid prescribing, increases in the number of providers allowed to prescribe buprenorphine, more syringe service programs to decrease needle sharing, improved naloxone access and increasing naloxone access to trained responders, and improved HCV screening and treatment programs. Although the indicators presented here share underlying causes and public health needs, individual indicators also suggest specific public health programmatic opportunities. For example, high HIV diagnoses in PWID suggest opportunities for scaling up pre-exposure prophylaxis among PWIDs, and prompt referral to HIV care and programs to support adherence in antiretroviral therapy care. High HCV diagnoses suggest opportunities for HCV treatment programs, coupled with harm reduction programs to prevent reinfection. For infectious disease physicians, awareness of the specific indicators that document OUD in their communities and states should influence the frequency of screening for infectious consequences of OUD and indicate the need for robust referral networks for specific types of prevention services outside of the clinical setting.

OUD is a complex health condition with a myriad of negative health outcomes. Given the complexity of addiction and the multiple forms of opioid misuse that occur, understanding OUD requires the triangulation of different data sources. Because different infectious disease surveillance systems have different strengths and weaknesses, ecological analyses can increase the sensitivity of a process of characterizing where services are needed compared with analysis of any single indicator. Moreover, more granular data are needed because available evidence indicates that there are subtle but important local differences in local populations, in the availability of local interventions, and in the types and routes of drugs used. Surveillance is the cornerstone of advocacy, awareness, and evidence-based public health response. We call for increased investments in multiple aspects of surveillance, especially for case-based surveillance for hepatitis C infection, and for sentinel surveillance activities to advance our understanding of how geographic characteristics of the epidemic play out at the level of people, rather than at the level of health jurisdictions.

REFERENCES

1. Peters PJ, Pontones P, Hoover KW, et al. HIV infection linked to injection use of oxymorphone in Indiana, 2014–2015. N Engl J Med 2016;375(3):229–39.
2. Rudd R, Aleshire N, Zibbell J, et al. Increases in drug and opioid overdose deaths—United States, 2000–2014. MMWR 2016;64(50):1378–82.
3. Han B, Compton WM, Blanco C, et al. Prescription Opioid Use, Misuse, and Use Disorders in U.S. Adults: 2015 National Survey on Drug Use and Health. Ann Intern Med 2017;167(5):293–301.
4. National Academies of Sciences, Engineering, and Medicine; Health and Medicine Division; Board on Population Health and Public Health Practice. Integrating responses at the intersection of opioid use disorder and infectious disease epidemics: proceedings of a workshop. Washington, DC: National Academies Press (US); 2018. p. 2. The Scope of the Problem. Available at: https://www.ncbi.nlm.nih.gov/books/NBK525643/.
5. Jones CM, McAninch JK. Emergency department visits and overdose deaths from combined use of opioids and benzodiazepines. Am J Prev Med 2015;49(4):493–501.
6. Rockett IR, Hobbs GR, Wu D, et al. Variable classification of drug-intoxication suicides across US states: a partial artifact of forensics? PLoS One 2015;10(8):e0135296.
7. Nakashima AK, Fleming PL. HIV/AIDS surveillance in the United States, 1981-2001. J Acquir Immune Defic Syndr 2003;32(Suppl 1):S68–85.
8. Centers for Disease Control and Prevention. NCHHSTP AtlasPlus [online data portal] 2019. Available at: https://www.cdc.gov/nchhstp/atlas/index.htm. Accessed September 2, 2019.
9. Valdiserri RO, Sullivan PS. Data visualization promotes sound public health practice: the AIDSvu example. AIDS Educ Prev 2018;30(1):26–34.
10. Centers for Disease Control and Prevention. Diagnoses of HIV Infection in the United States and Dependent Areas, 2017; vol. 29. 2018. Available at: http://www.cdc.gov/hiv/library/reports/surveillance/index.html. Accessed March 17, 2019.
11. New York Department Health. New York State HIV/AIDS Annual Surveillance Report. 2019. Available at: https://www.health.ny.gov/diseases/aids/general/statistics/annual/2018/2018_annual_surveillance_report.pdf. Accessed: April 24, 2020.

12. Bradley H, Hall EW, Rosenthal EM, et al. Hepatitis C Virus Prevalence in 50 US States and DC by Sex, Birth Cohort, and Race: 2013-2016. Hepatol Commun 2019;4(3):355–70.

13. Rosenberg ES, Hall EW, Sullivan PS, et al. Estimation of state-level prevalence of hepatitis C Virus Infection, US States and District of Columbia, 2010. Clin Infect Dis 2017;64(11):1573–81.

14. Rosenberg ES, Rosenthal EM, Hall EW, et al. Prevalence of Hepatitis C Virus Infection in US States and the District of Columbia, 2013 to 2016. JAMA Netw open 2018;1(8):e186371.

15. Centers for Disease Control and Prevention. WONDER [online data portal] 2019. Available at: http://wonder.cdc.gov. Accessed February 15, 2020.

16. Slavova S, O'Brien DB, Creppage K, et al. Drug overdose deaths: let's get specific. Public Health Rep 2015;130(4):339–42.

17. Lansky A, Abdul-Quader AS, Cribbin M, et al. Developing an HIV Behavioral Surveillance System for injecting drug users: the National HIV Behavioral Surveillance System. Public Health Rep 2007;122:48–55.

18. Centers for Disease Control and Prevention. HIV infection risk, prevention, and testing behaviors among persons who inject drugs—national HIV behavioral surveillance: injection drug use, 23 U.S. Cities, 2018. [online surveillance report]. HIV Surveillance Special Report 24. 2020. Available at: http://www.cdc.gov/hiv/library/reports/hivsurveillance.html. Accessed April 24, 2020.

19. Patel P, Borkowf CB, Brooks JT, et al. Estimating per-act HIV transmission risk: a systematic review. AIDS 2014;28(10):1509.

20. Evans ME, Labuda SM, Hogan V, et al. Notes from the field: HIV infection investigation in a rural area - West Virginia, 2017. MMWR Morb Mortal Wkly Rep 2018;67(8):257–8.

21. Cranston K, Alpren C, John B, et al. Notes from the Field: HIV Diagnoses Among Persons Who Inject Drugs—Northeastern Massachusetts, 2015–2018. MMWR Morb Mortal Wkly Rep 2019;68(10):253.

22. Chen WJ, Fang C-C, Shyu R-S, et al. Underreporting of illicit drug use by patients at emergency departments as revealed by two-tiered urinalysis. Addict behaviors 2006;31(12):2304–8.

23. Sowell RL, Lowenstein A, Moneyham L, et al. Resources, stigma, and patterns of disclosure in rural women with HIV infection. Public Health Nurs 1997;14(5):302–12.

24. Luoma JB, Twohig MP, Waltz T, et al. An investigation of stigma in individuals receiving treatment for substance abuse. Addict behaviors 2007;32(7):1331–46.

25. Day C, Conroy E, Lowe J, et al. Patterns of drug use and associated harms among rural injecting drug users: comparisons with metropolitan injecting drug users. Aust J Rural Health 2006;14(3):120–5.

26. CDC. Viral Hepatitis Surveillance, United States 2017. [online surveillance report] 2019. Available at: https://www.cdc.gov/hepatitis/statistics/2017surveillance/pdfs/2017HepSurveillanceRpt.pdf. Accessed: April 24, 2020.

27. Hutchinson SJ, Bird SM, Taylor A, et al. Modelling the spread of hepatitis C virus infection among injecting drug users in Glasgow: implications for prevention. Int J Drug Policy 2006;17(3):211–21.

28. Corson S, Greenhalgh D, Taylor A, et al. Modelling the prevalence of HCV amongst people who inject drugs: an investigation into the risks associated with injecting paraphernalia sharing. Drug Alcohol Depend 2013;133(1):172–9.

29. Van Handel MM, Rose CE, Hallisey EJ, et al. County-Level Vulnerability Assessment for Rapid Dissemination of HIV or HCV Infections Among Persons Who Inject Drugs, United States. J Acquir Immune Defic Syndr 2016;73(3):323–31.

30. Ramachandran S, Thai H, Forbi JC, et al. A large HCV transmission network enabled a fast-growing HIV outbreak in rural Indiana, 2015. EBioMedicine 2018;37:374–81.

31. Abara WE, Trujillo L, Broz D, et al. Age-related differences in past or present hepatitis C virus infection among people who inject drugs: national human immunodeficiency virus behavioral surveillance, 8 US Cities, 2015. J Infect Dis 2019; 220(3):377–85.

32. amFAR. Opioid & Health Indicators Database [online data repository]. 2020. Available at: https://opioid.amfar.org/. Accessed: April 24: 2020.

33. Singer M, Himmelgreen D, Dushay R, et al. Variation in drug injection frequency among out-of-treatment drug users in a national sample. Am J Drug Alcohol Abuse 1998;24(2):321–41.

34. Hedergaard H, Minino AM, Warner M. Drug overdose deaths in the United States, 1999–2018 – NCHS data brief No. 356. [online data report] 2020. Available at: https://www.cdc.gov/nchs/products/databriefs/db356.htm. Accessed: April 24, 2020.

35. Centers for Disease Control and Prevention. U.S. Opioid Prescribing Rate Maps [online data report[. 2020. Available at: https://www.cdc.gov/drugoverdose/maps/rxrate-maps.html. Accessed: April 24, 2020.

36. Guy GP Jr, Zhang K, Bohm MK, et al. Vital signs: changes in opioid prescribing in the United States, 2006–2015. MMWR Morb Mortal Wkly Rep 2017;66(26):697.

37. Scholl L, Seth P, Kariisa M, et al. Drug and opioid-involved overdose deaths—United States, 2013–2017. MMWR Morb Mortal Wkly Rep 2019;67(5152):1419.

38. Kolodny A, Courtwright DT, Hwang CS, et al. The prescription opioid and heroin crisis: a public health approach to an epidemic of addiction. Annu Rev Public Health 2015;36:559–74.

39. Rudd RA, Aleshire N, Zibbell JE, et al. Increases in drug and opioid overdose deaths—United States, 2000–2014. Am J Transplant 2016;16(4):1323–7.

40. Centers for Disease Control and Prevention. CDC Wonder 2018 [online public health data portal]. Available at https://wonder.cdc.gov/ucd-icd10.html. Accessed April 9, 2020.

41. Centers for Disease Control and Prevention. 2018 Annual Surveillance Report of Drug-Related Risks and Outcomes — United States. [Surveillance Special Report]. 2018. Available at: https://www.cdc.gov/drugoverdose/pdf/pubs/2018-cdc-drug-surveillance-report.pdf. Accessed April 24, 2020.

42. Seth P, Rudd RA, Noonan RK, et al. Quantifying the epidemic of prescription opioid overdose deaths. J American Public Health Association 2018;108:500–2.

43. Tote KM, Bradley H, Martin EG, et al. Factors associated with incomplete toxicology reporting in drug overdose deaths, 2010–2016. Ann Epidemiol 2019; 38:65–9.

44. Lowder EM, Ray BR, Huynh P, et al. Identifying unreported opioid deaths through toxicology data and vital records linkage: case study in Marion County, Indiana, 2011-2016. Am J Public Health 2018;108(12):1682–7.

45. Warner M, Hedegaard H. Identifying opioid overdose deaths using vital statistics data. Am J Public Health 2018;108(12):1587–9.

46. Laing MK, Tupper KW, Fairbairn N. Drug checking as a potential strategic overdose response in the fentanyl era. Int J Drug Policy 2018;62:59–66.

47. McClellan C, Lambdin BH, Ali MM, et al. Opioid-overdose laws association with opioid use and overdose mortality. Addict behaviors 2018;86:90–5.

48. Dunne RB. Prescribing naloxone for opioid overdose intervention. Pain Manag 2018;8(3):197–208.

49. Rigg KK, Monnat SM, Chavez MN. Opioid-related mortality in rural America: geographic heterogeneity and intervention strategies. Int J Drug Policy 2018; 57:119–29.

50. Piantadosi S, Byar DP, Green SB. The ecological fallacy. Am J Epidemiol 1988; 127(5):893–904.

51. Gallagher KM, Sullivan PS, Lansky A, et al. Behavioral surveillance among people at risk for HIV infection in the U.S.: the National HIV Behavioral Surveillance System. Public Health Rep 2007;122(Suppl 1):32–8.

52. Lansky A, Sullivan PS, Gallagher KM, et al. HIV behavioral surveillance in the US: a conceptual framework. Public Health Rep 2007;122(1_suppl):16–23.

53. McNaghten AD, Wolfe MI, Onorato I, et al. Improving the representativeness of behavioral and clinical surveillance for persons with HIV in the United States: the rationale for developing a population-based approach. PLoS One 2007; 2(6):e550.

54. Centers for Disease Control and Prevention. STD Surveillance network SSuN. [online surveillance system description]. 2020. Available at: https://www.cdc.gov/std/ssun/default.htm. Accessed: April 25, 2020.

55. Rietmeijer CA, Donnelly J, Bernstein KT, et al. Here comes the SSuN: early experiences with the STD Surveillance Network. Public Health Rep 2009; 124(2_suppl):72–7.

56. National Institutes of Health. Helping to End Addiction Long-term. [online program description]. 2017. Available at: https://www.hhs.gov/hepatitis/blog/2017/09/06/grants-awarded-to-address-opioid-crisis-in-rural-regions.html. Accessed: April 25, 2020.

57. Monnat SM, Peters DJ, Berg MT, et al. Using census data to understand county-level differences in overall drug mortality and opioid-related mortality by opioid type. Am J Public Health 2019;109(8):1084–91.

58. Monnat SM. Factors associated with county-level differences in U.S. drug-related mortality rates. Am J Prev Med 2018;54(5):611–9.

59. Nosrati E, Kang-Brown J, Ash M, et al. Economic decline, incarceration, and mortality from drug use disorders in the USA between 1983 and 2014: an observational analysis. Lancet Public Health 2019;4(7):e326–33.

60. Haffajee RL, Lin LA, Bohnert ASB, et al. Characteristics of US counties with high opioid overdose mortality and low capacity to deliver medications for opioid use disorder. JAMA Netw open 2019;2(6):e196373.

61. Keyes KM, Cerdá M, Brady JE, et al. Understanding the rural-urban differences in nonmedical prescription opioid use and abuse in the United States. Am J Public Health 2014;104(2):e52–9.

62. Centers for Disease Control and Prevention. Enhanced State Opioid Overdose Surveillance [online program description]. 2020. Available at: https://www.cdc.gov/drugoverdose/foa/state-opioid-mm.html. Accessed: April 27, 2020.

The Clinical Microbiology Laboratory and the Opioid Epidemic: Challenges and Opportunities

Simeon D. Kimmel, MD, MA[a,b],*, Nancy S. Miller, MD[c]

KEYWORDS

• Microbiology laboratory • Opioid crisis • Injection drug associated infections

KEY POINTS

- Increasing numbers of infections associated with injection drug use present new challenges for the diagnostic microbiology laboratory.
- The microbiology laboratory would benefit from additional resources, protocol revisions, and improved clinical communication to serve the increased clinical needs associated with injection drug related infections.
- The microbiology laboratory is an important partner for clinicians and the public health system to improve care for patients with injection drug associated infections.

INTRODUCTION

Increasing injection drug use amidst the opioid crisis has led to dramatic increases in injection drug use -associated infections, including serious bacterial infections and viral infections.[1–9] These infections reflect a complex mix of contributory factors, simultaneously social, political, behavioral, and microbiological: Injection and drug use behaviors, harm reduction and addiction treatment access and practices, host immune status, and specific complications caused by tissue-tropic and toxigenic pathogens.[10–15] For people who inject drugs (PWID), the risk of infection is high, the range

Both authors contributed equally to this article.
a Section of Infectious Diseases, Department of Medicine, Boston Medical Center, Boston University School of Medicine, 72 East Concord Street, Boston, MA 02118, USA; b Section of General Internal Medicine, Department of Medicine, Boston Medical Center, Boston University School of Medicine, 72 East Concord Street, Boston, MA 02118, USA; c Department of Pathology and Laboratory Medicine, Boston Medical Center, Boston University School of Medicine, 670 Albany Street, Suite 733, Boston, MA 02118, USA
* Corresponding author. Sections of Infectious Diseases and General Internal Medicine, 801 Massachusetts Avenue, Crosstown Building, 2nd Floor, Boston, MA 02118.
E-mail address: Simeon.Kimmel@bmc.org

Infect Dis Clin N Am 34 (2020) 465–478
https://doi.org/10.1016/j.idc.2020.06.005
0891-5520/20/© 2020 Elsevier Inc. All rights reserved.

id.theclinics.com

of infections is broad, and the complications can be life threatening. Infections among PWID can be exacerbated by interruptions in care with resulting escalation of clinical acuity, partial treatment, and potential for antimicrobial resistance.[16–18] Too few PWID receive treatment for their underlying addiction or are linked with evidence-based harm reduction strategies when they come into care for infectious complications of substance use.[19–21] Infection-related morbidity is then exacerbated by attritional adverse effects of substance use on overall medical, social, and economic stability.[10,22–26]

Injection practices including frequency and sharing, type of drug injected, use of sterile syringes, and skin cleaning and preparation, as well as risk from contaminated drugs, solvents and equipment, all have important implications for risk and type of infections.[11,12,27] There is a broad range of injection drug–associated infections from aerobic and anaerobic mucocutaneous commensals, toxin producers, agents of sexually transmitted infections, and opportunistic pathogens including water and soil species (**Tables 1** and **2**). PWID are at risk for localized and disseminated infections include osteomyelitis, skin and soft tissue infections, endophthalmitis, brain and other parenchymal abscesses, bacteremias, infective endocarditis, and sterile body fluid infections.[6,10,13,28–30]

The public health and clinical systems are responding to the opioid crisis with new programs and initiatives to address the rising morbidity and mortality. A variety of approaches are being used, including reduction of opioid prescribing, delivery of medication for opioid use disorder through addiction consult services and low-barrier buprenorphine clinics, integration of harm reduction services into clinical services, and expansion of community and pharmacy naloxone. These efforts have all required additional staffing and resources to meet the needs of people who use opioids and other drugs.[31–37] Similarly, the diagnostic microbiology laboratory must respond in support of these patients and the clinicians who care for them. In doing so, many challenges have emerged despite recent advances in diagnostic technologies and laboratory practices. In this review, we present clinical vignettes that illustrate less recognized and unique challenges that the microbiology laboratory may confront amid the ongoing opioid crisis, despite limitations in personnel and financial resources. These factors include a broad spectrum of usual and unusual pathogens, technological limitations, protocols, and policies and regulatory requirements not designed with PWID in mind, as well as an increased need for collaboration and communication with key stakeholders.

Table 1
Injection drug use associated infections and related morbidities

Infections	Related Morbidities
Bacteremia	Acute-on-chronic infections
Sepsis	Partially treated infections
Endocarditis	Antimicrobial resistance
Skin and soft tissue, abscesses	Repeated admissions
Necrotizing fasciitis, pyogenic myositis	Interruptions in care
Toxic shock syndrome	Interim escalation of clinical acuity
Wound botulism and tetanus	Extended hospital length of stay
Pneumonia	Social and economic health adversities
Osteomyelitis, septic arthritis	
Septic thrombophlebitis, venous sclerosis	
HIV, other sexually transmitted diseases, hepatitis, *Mycobacterium tuberculosis*	
Disseminated, polymicrobial infections	

Table 2	
Injection drug use: increased risk, potential pathogens[1]	
Staphylococcus aureus	Mycobacterium tuberculosis, other acid-fast bacilli
Pathogenic streptococci	
Opportunistic strep, strep-like species	Actinomyces species
Salmonella, other Enterobacteriaceae	Nocardia species
Pseudomonas aeruginosa	Legionella pneumophila
Opportunistic nonenteric gram-negative rods	Candida species yeast
	Herpes simplex virus
Eikenella, Capnocytophaga	Toxoplasma gondii
Fusobacterium species	Treponema pallidum, other sexually transmitted diseases
Clostridium, Bacillus, Lactobacillus	
Listeria monocytogenes	HIV
Other aerobic and anaerobic flora	Hepatitis A, B, and C viruses
	Free-living ameba

From Kaushik et al Kapila K, Praharaj AK. Shooting up: The interface of microbial infections and drug abuse. *J Med Microbiol.* 2011;60(4):408-422 and Gordon RJ, Lowy FD. Bacterial infections in drug users. *N Engl J Med.* 2005;353(18):1945-1954; with permission.

CLINICAL SCENARIOS
Staphylococcus aureus

Case 1
A patient who injects drugs is found to have high-grade methicillin-susceptible *Staphylococcus aureus* bacteremia with concern for embolic infective endocarditis.

Case 2
A patient who injects drugs is found to have high-grade methicillin-resistant *S aureus* (MRSA) also with concern for embolic infective endocarditis.

Challenges to the laboratory

1. Test volume
2. Resources
3. Technological limitations
4. Laboratory protocols.

Infective endocarditis is a dreaded complication of injection drug use with substantial resulting mortality and morbidity.[20,38,39] These costly infections have dramatically increased amid the opioid crisis. Infective endocarditis typically requires prolonged courses of intravenous antibiotics and frequently cardiac valve replacement surgery.[40,41] High-grade, persistent bacteremias associated with infective endocarditis have significant implications for the microbiology laboratory in several ways. The increased volume of blood and other cultures stress the laboratory workflow. Because PWID may present variably and with limited early manifestations of infective endocarditis, there may be need for both several initial blood cultures and subsequent serial blood cultures to monitor clearance of bacteremia, important both to determine treatment efficacy and also duration of therapy. Injection-associated local and disseminated infections may result in additional nonvascular site cultures necessary for both diagnosis and management (skin, soft tissue, bone, and parenchyma).[40,41] Laboratory staff must be trained to understand the clinical reasons for serial cultures and their clinical usefulness to ensure that the samples are processed and referenced appropriately. For example, laboratory policies must address referral protocols, that is, how many individual positive blood culture results are called as a critical action value (requiring a cascade of communication with the clinical team); how many results will be referred to a prior blood culture without evaluation of the susceptibility patterns of an individual isolate and for what duration. Referral protocols may differ for laboratories using only culture-based methods versus those who also rely on molecular and/ or proteomic testing such as matrix-assisted laser desorption/ionization-time of flight mass spectrometry (MALDI-TOF MS) and other methods for microbiological profiling, including identification and resistance markers such as the mecA gene for MRSA.

Additionally, protocol triggers may be required for troubleshooting and subsequent testing for these isolates. For example, the laboratory must address serial cultures that alternate between MRSA and methicillin-susceptible *Staphylococcus aureus* and determine protocols for susceptibility testing for antibiotic alternatives to vancomycin when the minimum inhibitory concentration (MIC) increases. Incorporating molecular testing into phenotypic blood culture workflow adds additional procedural complexity. The laboratory must negotiate discrepant molecular results or molecular results that are different from culture-derived results. Additionally, the laboratory must be attentive to correlation between blood cultures and culture results from other sites.[42] Routine laboratory workflow may already address these considerations. However, the increased number of cultures and complexity of testing specific to PWID notably stresses existing infrastructure and may require modifications to usual routine.

Bacillus Species

Case 3
An adult patient who had been injecting drugs was admitted with sepsis. He was found to have disseminated MRSA bacteremia. A large beta-hemolytic, catalase-positive gram-positive rod was recovered from the aerobic bottle of 1 of 2 admission blood culture sets. The organism was identified by MALDI-TOF MS as belonging to the *Bacillus cereus* group. *Bacillus anthracis*, another *B cereus* group species, was ruled out by beta-hemolysis and colonial morphology.

Case 4
An adult patient who had been injecting drugs was admitted with pneumonia and sepsis. Blood cultures recovered a Bacillus-like species that was nonhemolytic and nonmotile. Owing to injection of drugs with contaminated equipment and soil exposure there was increased concern for *Bacillus* infection. Owing to the risk for *B anthracis* and potential anthracis variants, a rule out-refer protocol was implemented.

Challenges to the laboratory

1. Resources
2. Protocols
3. Expertise
4. Communication

Bacillus species are zoonotic, environmental and spore-forming gram-positive bacilli. Bacillus infections, including anthrax, have long been associated with injection drug use. But *B cereus* bacteremias are increasingly reported in persons who inject drugs owing to its role as a skin commensal and contaminant of drug and injection equipment. *B cereus* infection among PWID can be atypical, and/or prolonged, serious infections.[43,44] Before the increasing numbers of infections associated with injection drug use, a single positive blood culture consistent with a non–anthracis *Bacillus* species, was considered a phlebotomy contaminant and additional identification and susceptibility testing was rarely warranted. Among PWID, however, the predictive clinical significance of these cultures is confounded by noncontiguous positive cultures, coinfection with *S aureus* and other recognized pathogens, partially treated infections, endocarditis, as well as phlebotomy challenges owing to venous scarring among PWID.[43–47]

MALDI-TOF MS offers faster, cost-effective database-dependent speciation with improved accuracy compared with traditional biochemical methods for those microbiology laboratories that have invested in this technology. Before using MALDI-TOF MS, careful phenotypic and even clinical correlation is advised to ensure proper biosafety during sample preparation and testing and to mitigate risk for misidentification between anthracis and non-anthracis species. For those isolates clearly non-anthracis *Bacillus* phenotypically, susceptibility testing may be even more important than speciation to ensure targeted antibiotic therapy and deescalation from empiric vancomycin. Deescalation, however, is challenged by unreliable susceptibility profiles for *B cereus* and *Bacillus thuringiensis*, another member of the *B cereus* group.[48,49]

Diagnostic laboratories providing services for PWID can anticipate an increase in the number of Bacillus species recovered in blood cultures. These isolates can no longer be immediately considered culture contaminants. For isolates consistent with a non-anthracis species, clinical correlation is imperative. MIC testing may be needed. Laboratories that do not perform requisite broth dilution testing to determine MICs may be faced with sending isolates to a reference laboratory. These additional "send out" tests tax the operating budgets and gatekeeping resources in microbiology laboratories and, importantly, increase time to actionable clinical results.

Nonhemolytic *Bacillus* species in cultures from PWID require proper evaluation and clinical correlation to rule out *B anthracis*. Underestimating the possibility of *B anthracis* poses biosafety risks in the laboratory including unprotected exposures and misidentification by methods unable to reliably distinguish *B anthracis* from other *B cereus* group species. Sentinel laboratories participating in the Laboratory Response Network follow a specific rule-out–refer protocol that requires suspect *B anthracis* isolate to be sent to a designated Laboratory Response Network reference laboratory (eg, a state public health laboratory) before any additional manipulations. In contrast, invoking a rule-out–refer protocol, where the isolate is sent to the Laboratory Response Network reference laboratory to exclude *B anthracis*, may delay isolate profiling.[50] To facilitate timely resolution of these cultures, it is imperative that a laboratory comply with biosafety protocols and have procedures that ensure escalation to supervisory or directorship oversight and communication with key stakeholders including the clinical care provider, and the Public Health and reference laboratories for referrals.

Clostridium Species

Case 5
A patient died after clostridial necrotizing myositis after injection drug use. Direct smears from wound tissue demonstrated myonecrosis with a dirty necrotic background, gas bubbles, a paucity of intact inflammatory cells, and abundant bacilli with variable staining.

Challenges to the laboratory

1. Expertise
2. Protocols
3. Communication
4. Technology

Clostridium species are spore-forming pathogens that frequently contaminate illicit drugs and injecting equipment. Facilitated by the heat resistance of bacterial spores, these pathogens can proliferate during drug preparation and in the favorable microenvironment of injection sites. A variety of species (including *C perfringens, C septicum,* and *C novyi,* among others) can cause skin and soft tissue infections. Other manifestations of clostridial infection include toxin-mediated wound botulism (*C botulinum*), tetanus (*C tetani*), and necrotizing fasciitis and myositis (*C perfringens,* other species), which have been especially associated with black tar heroin.[47] Although severe necrotizing infections may be recognized clinically, the laboratory staff must be educated to recognize the potential significance of such findings during direct smear examination in conjunction with culture evaluation and clinical correlation. Like Bacillus species, diagnostic laboratories are additionally challenged by the resources and expertise necessary for anaerobic culture and accurate identification of clostridial species.

Unexpected and Unidentified Findings

Case 6
A person presented with systemic infection after injecting drugs. Before injection, the patient reported licking the needle that was used to administer the drugs. Blood cultures recovered thin gram-positive bacilli without spores that were not identified by direct target-based multiplex polymerase chain reaction from an aliquot of the positive blood culture. The clinical team changed empiric therapy from vancomycin to ampicillin-sulbactam owing to the Gram stain results after discussion with microbiology laboratory staff. A Lactobacillus species was identified by culture and confirmed by MALDI-TOF MS the following day. Notably, *Lactobacillus* species were not included in the database of the multiplex polymerase chain reaction assay.

Case 7
A young adult presented with chills, dyspnea, and bloody cough after injecting drugs. The patient's past medical includes high-grade methicillin-susceptible *Staphylococcus aureus* endocarditis with septic emboli and numerous disruptions in care. Filamentous gram-positive rods were recovered in 1 of 3 initial blood cultures after 4 days of incubation. Further testing demonstrated these this isolate was modified acid fast positive, catalase positive, and nonpigmented. The isolate was subsequently identified as a *Streptomyces* species by DNA sequencing at a reference laboratory after in-house phenotypic methods and MALDI-TOF MS proteomics failed to provide identification.

Case 8
An adult with a history of injection drug use presented with mitral valve endocarditis that required valve replacement. A culture of the native valve recovered a yeast-like fungus identified by reference laboratory DNA sequencing as the plant smut (mold) *Tilletiopsis albescens.* We were not aware of previously reported human infections for *T albescens.* Notably, a cousin species *T minor* has been implicated in 2 reports of serious infection in a setting of immunocompromise.[51,52]

Challenges to the laboratory

1. Expertise
2. Resources
3. Technology
4. Communication
5. Quality metrics

The cases presented challenge the microbiology laboratory and infectious disease clinicians to ascribe clinical significance to microbiological findings. The isolates in cases 7 and 8 may not be truly implicated in the underlying clinical presentations, but PWID may present with alarming symptoms and noncontiguous positive blood cultures that may yield a variety of environmental organisms that can no longer be dismissed a priori as clinically insignificant. Lactobacilli, for example, are opportunistic pathogens that have been reported in association with serious cases of bacteremias and/or infective endocarditis in PWID and patients who do not inject drugs.[53–56] Several aerotolerant *Lactobacillus* species are intrinsically vancomycin resistant and some have variable resistance to penicillins and cephalosporins.[55,56] Therefore, prompt identification in cultures from PWID is important to clinical management, especially after a suspect Gram stain raises the possibility of lactobacilli. However, susceptibility testing for lactobacilli, like *Bacillus* species, requires broth dilution MIC method that may be beyond the reach of routine laboratories without reliance on a reference laboratory.[49]

Additionally, these cases highlight the limitations of commercial target-based and database-dependent technologies used by routine diagnostic laboratories. US Food and Drug Administration–cleared systems often do not include species relevant to injection drug microbiology, especially those that are uncommon or environmental and considered unlikely to be clinically relevant. Off-label verifications can be performed to extend the usefulness of some US Food and Drug Administration–cleared in vitro diagnostic systems. However, this approach may be beyond a routine laboratory's budget and expertise. Subsequently, the laboratory must rely on costly and time-consuming reference laboratory resources.

The cases presented in this article highlight the challenge of differentiating positive blood cultures that represent true clinical infections from laboratory contaminants. Although this has obvious clinical implications, the increase in positive *Lactobacillus* and *Bacillus* blood cultures also complicate the quality reporting for microbiology laboratories. Quality metrics for microbiology laboratories include blood culture contamination rates. So-called initial specimen diversion devices may decrease blood culture contamination at the time of phlebotomy draw and allow clinically significant commensals to be more easily interpreted as such. These devices require strategic investment of resources if a laboratory can offset the additional cost by downstream savings. However, to ensure quality measures are appropriately applied, current algorithms require revision to exclude clinically significant *Bacillus* or other atypical pathogens, or at minimum, adjustment for a patient population with high rates of injection drug use. Changes in pathogen recovery rates over time linked to clinical data can be used to indicate if changes are associated with increased injection drug use in an institution's patient population.

Human Immunodeficiency Virus, Hepatis C Virus, and Syphilis

Case 9
A young man who injects heroin, fentanyl, cocaine, and methamphetamine and reports sharing injection equipment as well as several episodes of transactional sex without use of barrier protection presents for human immunodeficiency virus (HIV), hepatitis C virus (HCV), and sexually transmitted infection screening. His last episode of unprotected sex and use of shared injection equipment was 48 hours ago.

Laboratory challenges

1. Expertise
2. Resources

3. Protocols
4. Collaboration
5. Quality management.

PWID have increased rates of transmissible HCV, HIV, and syphilis, all of which currently require algorithmic testing using different assays and specimen types. As clinicians increase efforts to deliver HIV pre-exposure and postexposure prophylaxis to people who use drugs and more protocols for rapid initiation of antiretroviral therapy for those with new diagnoses of HIV, timely and complete testing is necessary. Microbiology laboratories have focused on ensuring reflex testing protocols so that closed-loop processes in which all components of the diagnostic algorithm are performed within a given center's laboratory to minimize delays and facilitate navigation to care. Laboratory results from these algorithms may require local expertise to assist with interpretation, engagement, and clinical management. In particular, the prompt resolution of HIV testing algorithms with HIV viral load testing are crucial to determining clinical management with pre-exposure or postexposure HIV prophylaxis. Similarly, rapid, closed-loop results for HCV antibody testing reflexes to viral load and genotype testing, which enables clinicians to more rapidly engage PWID with active HCV infection in treatment with direct-acting antivirals. Syphilis testing, with variable strategies by center, requires collaboration with departments of public health and clinicians to interpret test results to ensure that patients receive appropriate treatment when necessary. To successfully implement these processes and interventions, support and coordination across various institutional stakeholders is required.[57]

CLINICIANS AND THE LABORATORIES: SHARED CHALLENGES

To optimally care for people with infectious compilations of injection drug use, coordination between clinicians and the diagnostic laboratory is paramount.[58] Key components of this relationship are mutual understanding, communication, and advocacy. Despite shared goals, clinical providers and laboratorians are not always well-versed in each other's practice and operational arenas. However, shared knowledge about pathogens and disease processes, clinical and laboratory workflows, and technological capacities enhances the clinical care provided to patients and the ability to subsequently improve workflow and protocols. Clinical and laboratory leadership should know each other well and collaborate on educational outreach and operational policies of mutual interest. Providers who most use the diagnostic laboratory (eg, infectious diseases, antimicrobial stewardship teams) should be familiar with front-line laboratory staff and laboratory protocols to facilitate communication and expectations. Strategies to forge and maintain these relationships includes orientation rotations in the laboratory for infectious disease and pharmacy fellows, serial didactic plate rounds and ad hoc team visits to the laboratory. Providers and laboratorians must both understand the challenges of providing expert yet cost-effective diagnostics so both parties may participate in effective advocacy for resources to support patient care.

As clinical services for PWID are developed in community settings, the need for collaboration and timely laboratory expertise and services will increase. The microbiology laboratory has an opportunity to support these efforts to meet the growing clinical need. Additionally, the laboratory may be the first place where new HIV resistance patterns or increases in certain types of infections are identified. Although microbiology laboratories have existing relationships with Departments of Public Health for specific reporting protocols,[59] there are opportunities to strengthen these efforts as it relates to the health of PWID.[60]

OPPORTUNITIES TO ADDRESS CHALLENGES IN THE MICROBIOLOGY LABORATORY AND IMPROVE SERVICES FOR PEOPLE WHO INJECTION DRUGS

The past decade has seen a notable increase in improved, user-friendly commercialized in-vitro diagnostics for infectious diseases, expanding the testing capability of routine laboratories. These technologies include a variety of target-based, sample-to-answer multiplexed molecular assays for pathogen detection and profiling directly from clinical specimens or after blood culture amplification. MALDI-TOF MS enables a broad range of proteomic microbial identifications from pure culture growth, with greater accuracy and shorter result times compared with traditional phenotypic methods. Automated high-throughput instruments dispatch molecular testing for viral load testing and sexually transmitted disease pathogen detection. Target-based detection of some bacterial and yeast species may now be performed directly from whole blood without culture. Some pathogen identification and MIC susceptibility testing from a positive blood culture is now possible within a laboratory shift. However, these technologies pose their own set of challenges. In their current incarnations, they are often additive to laboratory costs and workflow because they cannot entirely replace traditional culture-based methods. Microbial profiling is hampered by target and database limitations inherent in the new methods. Automated susceptibility testing still suffers from lack of protocol flexibility, technical limitations, and suboptimal time to results. Electronic laboratory and information technology systems have not optimally adjusted to keep pace with the complexities of integrated data management and result reporting owing to changes in diagnostic technology and laboratory practices.

Increasing numbers of infections owing to injection drug use amid the opioid epidemic has magnified these areas of laboratory practice that remain challenged despite advances in technology. We suggest several improvements that could enable the laboratory to better meet the clinical needs of PWID and address these challenges (**Box 1**). First, laboratory budgets are taxed owing to increased test volume and complexity, which require increased human, technological, and financial resources. For laboratories to respond to this important public health crisis, additional investments may be necessary. Microbiology laboratories require resources to develop new expertise and technical capacity in response to the HIV epidemic and the same is true now. Respective professional organizations can be leveraged to lobby for increased support of public health infrastructure. Laboratory and clinical stakeholders should support each other in bringing awareness of these issues to their institutional leadership. Second, we propose additional suggestions that could improve the diagnostic certainty, laboratory processes, and immediacy of treatment. Many of these suggestions require investments from companies who develop and commercialize in vitro diagnostics. The microbiological peculiarities of pathogens more common among PWID is a concept that may not gain traction in the pipeline of commercial in vitro diagnostics. However, laboratories need in vitro diagnostics platforms with flexible, dual-purpose applications directed to multiple patient populations. For example, broader and more flexible microbiological profiling and drug susceptibility testing could have allowed for timelier, in-house laboratory data in several of the presented cases. Novel technologies may be necessary to address this challenge to have it be a palatable investment for commercial enterprises. These suggestions could strengthen a laboratory's diagnostic and workflow efficiencies to optimize patient care. Although some solutions may be within reach, others require more time and investment. In the interim, these patient care challenges remain for laboratories, clinical providers, and health care facilities.

Box 1
Opportunities to mitigate challenges and improve diagnostics in the microbiology laboratory

1. Additional resources and investments.

2. Improved clinical data management systems that integrate results from multiple diagnostic methods, better integrate reflex testing, reporting results from repeat testing, discrepant resolution, and critical value documentation.

3. Direct interrogation of more specimen types with expanded pathogen detection capability (including fungal organisms).

4. Automated commercial systems that provide susceptibility testing for esoteric broth-based MIC protocols (eg, CLSI M-45).

5. US Food and Drug Administration–cleared commercialized, fully automated sample to answer sequencing technologies for microbiological profiling.

6. A cost-effective flexible approach to user-defined formularies for automated susceptibility testing.

7. A one and done approach to diagnostics for HIV, HCV, and syphilis: One-step definitive diagnostics to replace algorithmic testing for each.

8. Affordable blood culture diversion devices to reduce contamination rates.

9. Improved use and validation of commercial database-dependent MALDI-TOF MS to reduce the burden on individual laboratories.

SUMMARY

Injection drug use has a profound impact on the clinical microbiology laboratory. PWID often present with high acuity, escalating complications, and a broad array of pathogens that result in diagnostic challenges. Timely and accurate information from the laboratory is crucial for clinical management. However, specific bloodstream infections have rendered usual blood culture protocols less useful. The increase in atypical bacteremias requires additional expert oversight and a reevaluation of workflow and protocols. Although the current technologies have aided workflow in the laboratory with more timely and broad diagnostics, there remain important limitations that require new solutions. Collaboration between clinical providers and the laboratory can help optimize in vitro diagnostic support for patient care.

DISCLOSURE

Dr S.D. Kimmel received support from the National Institute on Drug Abuse (NIDA) (R25DA013582, R25DA033211), and the National Institute of Allergy and Infectious Diseases (5T32AI052074). He consults for Abt Associates on a Massachusetts Department of Public Health project to expand access to medications for opioid use disorder in postacute medical care facilities. Dr N.S. Miller reports support from the Massachusetts Department of Public Health (HIV/HCV/STI/TB Prevention, Linkage, and Retention in Care and Treatment Program).

REFERENCES

1. Ronan MV, Herzig SJ. Hospitalizations related to opioid abuse/dependence and associated serious infections increased sharply, 2002–12. Health Aff 2016;35(5): 832–7.
2. Peters PJ, Pontones P, Hoover KW, et al. HIV infection linked to injection use of oxymorphone in Indiana, 2014–2015. N Engl J Med 2016;375(3):229–39.

3. Cranston K, Alpren C, John B, et al. Notes from the field: HIV diagnoses among persons who inject drugs - Northeastern Massachusetts, 2015-2018. MMWR Morb Mortal Wkly Rep 2019;68(10):253–4.
4. Deo SV, Raza S, Kalra A, et al. Admissions for infective endocarditis in intravenous drug users. J Am Coll Cardiol 2018;71(14):1596–7.
5. Schranz AJ, Fleischauer A, Chu VH, et al. Trends in drug use-associated infective endocarditis and heart valve surgery, 2007 to 2017: a study of statewide discharge data. Ann Intern Med 2019;170(1):31–40.
6. Jackson KA, Bohm MK, Brooks JT, et al. Invasive methicillin-resistant staphylococcus aureus infections among persons who inject drugs - six sites, 2005-2016. MMWR Morb Mortal Wkly Rep 2018;67(22):625–8.
7. Suryaprasad AG, White JZ, Xu F, et al. Emerging epidemic of hepatitis C virus infections among young nonurban persons who inject drugs in the United States, 2006–2012. Clin Infect Dis 2014;59(10):1411–9.
8. Ciccarone D, Unick GJ, Cohen JK, et al. Nationwide increase in hospitalizations for heroin-related soft tissue infections: associations with structural market conditions. Drug Alcohol Depend 2016;163:126–33.
9. Zibbell JE, Iqbal K, Patel RC, et al. Increases in hepatitis C virus infection related to injection drug use among persons aged ≤30 years - Kentucky, Tennessee, Virginia, and West Virginia, 2006-2012. MMWR Morb Mortal Wkly Rep 2015;64(17): 453–8. Available at: http://www.ncbi.nlm.nih.gov/pubmed/25950251. Accessed October 7, 2019.
10. Gordon RJ, Lowy FD. Bacterial infections in drug users. N Engl J Med 2005; 353(18):1945–54.
11. Bluthenthal RN, Anderson R, Flynn NM, et al. Higher syringe coverage is associated with lower odds of HIV risk and does not increase unsafe syringe disposal among syringe exchange program clients. Drug Alcohol Depend 2007;89(2–3): 214–22.
12. Lambdin BH, Bluthenthal RN, Zibbell JE, et al. Associations between perceived illicit fentanyl use and infectious disease risks among people who inject drugs. Int J Drug Policy 2019. https://doi.org/10.1016/j.drugpo.2019.10.004.
13. Ciccarone D, Harris M. Fire in the vein: heroin acidity and its proximal effect on users' health. Int J Drug Policy 2015;26(11):1103–10.
14. Gostin LO, Hodge JG, Gulinson CL. Supervised injection facilities: legal and policy reforms. JAMA 2019;321(8):812.
15. Potier C, Laprévote V, Dubois-Arber F, et al. Supervised injection services: what has been demonstrated? A systematic literature review. Drug Alcohol Depend 2014;145:48–68.
16. Simon R, Snow R, Wakeman S. Understanding why patients with substance use disorders leave the hospital against medical advice: a qualitative study. Subst Abus 2019. https://doi.org/10.1080/08897077.2019.1671942.
17. Ti L, Ti L. Leaving the hospital against medical advice among people who use illicit drugs: a systematic review. Am J Public Health 2015;105(12). https://doi.org/10.2105/AJPH.2015.302885.
18. Southern WN, Nahvi S, Arnsten JH. Increased risk of mortality and readmission among patients discharged against medical advice. Am J Med 2012;125(6): 594–602.
19. Rosenthal ES, Karchmer AW, Theisen-Toupal J, et al. Suboptimal addiction interventions for patients hospitalized with injection drug use-associated infective endocarditis. Am J Med 2016;129(5):481–5.

20. Rodger L, Glockler-Lauf SD, Shojaei E, et al. Clinical characteristics and factors associated with mortality in first-episode infective endocarditis among persons who inject drugs. JAMA Netw Open 2018;1(7):e185220.
21. Vold JH, Aas C, Leiva RA, et al. Integrated care of severe infectious diseases to people with substance use disorders; a systematic review. BMC Infect Dis 2019; 19(1):306.
22. Haight SC, Ko JY, Van Tong VT, et al. Opioid use disorder documented at delivery hospitalization — United States, 1999–2014. Morb Mortal Wkly Rep 2018;67(31): 845–9.
23. Spaulding AC, Seals RM, Page MJ, et al. HIV/AIDS among inmates of and relea-sees from US correctional facilities, 2006: declining share of epidemic but persis-tent public health opportunity. PLoS One 2009;4(11):e7558.
24. Binswanger IA, Blatchford PJ, Mueller SR, et al. Mortality after prison release: opioid overdose and other causes of death, risk factors, and time trends from 1999 to 2009. Ann Intern Med 2013;159(9). https://doi.org/10.7326/0003-4819-159-9-201311050-00005.
25. Green TC, Clarke J, Brinkley-Rubinstein L, et al. Postincarceration fatal overdoses after implementing medications for addiction treatment in a statewide correc-tional system. JAMA Psychiatry 2018;75(4):405.
26. Somerville NJ, O'Donnell J, Gladden RM, et al. Characteristics of fentanyl over-dose - Massachusetts, 2014-2016. MMWR Morb Mortal Wkly Rep 2017;66(14): 382–6.
27. Vlahov D, Junge B, Brookmeyer R, et al. Reductions in high-risk drug use behav-iors among participants in the Baltimore needle exchange program. J Acquir Im-mune Defic Syndr Hum Retrovirol 1997;16(5):400–6. Available at: http://www.ncbi.nlm.nih.gov/pubmed/9420320. Accessed October 15, 2019.
28. Jafari S, Joe R, Elliot D, et al. A community care model of intravenous antibiotic therapy for injection drug users with deep tissue infection for "Reduce leaving against medical advice. Int J Ment Health Addict 2014;13(1). https://doi.org/10.1007/s11469-014-9511-4.
29. Larney S, Peacock A, Mathers BM, et al. A systematic review of injecting-related injury and disease among people who inject drugs. Drug Alcohol Depend 2017; 171. https://doi.org/10.1016/j.drugalcdep.2016.11.029.
30. Nagar VR, Springer JE, Salles S. Increased Incidence of Spinal Abscess and Substance Abuse after Implementation of State Mandated Prescription Drug Legislation. Pain Med 2015;16(10):2031–5.
31. Sharma M, Lamba W, Cauderella A, et al. Harm reduction in hospitals. Harm Re-duct J 2017;14(1):32.
32. Trowbridge P, Weinstein ZM, Kerensky T, et al. Addiction consultation services - Linking hospitalized patients to outpatient addiction treatment. J Subst Abuse Treat 2017;79:1–5.
33. Suzuki J. Medication-assisted treatment for hospitalized patients with intravenous-drug-use related infective endocarditis. Am J Addict 2016;25(3): 191–4.
34. Wakeman SE, Metlay JP, Chang Y, et al. Inpatient addiction consultation for hos-pitalized patients increases post-discharge abstinence and reduces addiction severity. J Gen Intern Med 2017;32(8):909–16.
35. Lim JK, Bratberg JP, Davis CS, et al. Prescribe to prevent: overdose prevention and naloxone rescue kits for prescribers and pharmacists. J Addict Med 2016; 10(5):300–8.

36. Walley AY, Xuan Z, Hackman HH, et al. Opioid overdose rates and implementation of overdose education and nasal naloxone distribution in Massachusetts: interrupted time series analysis. BMJ 2013;346:f174.
37. Saloner B, McGinty EE, Beletsky L, et al. A Public Health Strategy for the Opioid Crisis. Public Health Rep 2018;133(1_suppl):24S–34S.
38. Bor DH, Woolhandler S, Nardin R, et al. Infective endocarditis in the U.S., 1998-2009: a nationwide study. PLoS One 2013;8(3):e60033.
39. Njoroge LW, Al-Kindi SG, Koromia GA, et al. Changes in the association of rising infective endocarditis with mortality in people who inject drugs. JAMA Cardiol 2018;3(8):779.
40. Baddour LM, Wilson WR, Bayer AS, et al. Infective endocarditis in adults: diagnosis, antimicrobial therapy, and management of complications: a scientific statement for healthcare professionals from the American Heart Association. Circulation 2015;132(15):1435–86.
41. Wang A, Gaca JG, Chu VH. Management considerations in infective endocarditis: a review. JAMA 2018;320(1):72–83.
42. Clinical and Laboratory Standards Institute. Principles and procedures for blood cultures; approved guideline (M47-A). Wayne, PA. 2007. Available at: www.clsi.org. Accessed January 21, 2020.
43. Powell AG, Crozier JE, Hodgson H, et al. A case of septicaemic anthrax in an intravenous drug user. BMC Infect Dis 2011;11(1):21.
44. Ikeda M, Yagihara Y, Tatsuno K, et al. Clinical characteristics and antimicrobial susceptibility of Bacillus cereus blood stream infections. Ann Clin Microbiol Antimicrob 2015;14(1):43.
45. Rudrik JT, Soehnlen MK, Perry MJ, et al. Safety and accuracy of matrix-assisted laser desorption ionization-time of flight mass spectrometry for identification of highly pathogenic organisms. J Clin Microbiol 2017;55(12):3513–29.
46. Van Veen SQ, Claas ECJ, Kuijper EJ. High-throughput identification of bacteria and yeast by matrix-assisted laser desorption ionization-time of flight mass spectrometry in conventional medical microbiology laboratories. J Clin Microbiol 2010; 48(3):900–7.
47. Kaushik KS, Kapila K, Praharaj AK. Shooting up: the interface of microbial infections and drug abuse. J Med Microbiol 2011;60(4):408–22.
48. Clark AE, Kaleta EJ, Arora A, et al. Matrix-assisted laser desorption ionization-time of flight mass spectrometry: a fundamental shift in the routine practice of clinical microbiology. Clin Microbiol Rev 2013;26(3):547–603.
49. Clinical and Laboratory Standards Institute. Methods for antimicrobial dilution and disk susceptibility testing of infrequently isolated or fastidious bacteria, 3rd edition (M45). Wayne, PA. Available at: www.clsi.org. Accessed January 21, 2020.
50. American Society for Microbiology. LRN sentinel level clinical laboratory protocols. Available at: https://www.asm.org/Articles/Policy/Laboratory-Response-Network-LRN-Sentinel-Level-C. Accessed January 21, 2020.
51. Wang QM, Begerow D, Groenewald M, et al. Multigene phylogeny and taxonomic revision of yeasts and related fungi in the Ustilaginomycotina. Stud Mycol 2015; 81:55–83.
52. Ramani R, Ramani A, Wong SJ. Rapid flow cytometric susceptibility testing of Candida albicans. J Clin Microbiol 1997;35(9):2320–4. Available at: http://www.ncbi.nlm.nih.gov/pubmed/9276410. Accessed January 21, 2020.
53. Goldstein EJC, Wurcel AG, Merchant EA, et al. Emerging and underrecognized complications of illicit drug use. Clin Infect Dis 2015;61(12):1840–9.

54. Verani DA, Carretto E, Bono L, et al. Lactobacillus casei endocarditis in an intravenous heroin drug addict: a case report. Funct Neurol 1993;8(5):355–7. Available at: http://www.ncbi.nlm.nih.gov/pubmed/8144063. Accessed January 30, 2020.
55. Slover CM. Lactobacillus: a review. Clin Microbiol Newsl 2008;30(4):23–7.
56. Salminen MK, Rautelin H, Tynkkynen S, et al. Lactobacillus bacteremia, species identification, and antimicrobial susceptibility of 85 blood isolates. Clin Infect Dis 2006;42(5):e35–44.
57. Calner P, Sperring H, Ruiz-Mercado G, et al. HCV screening, linkage to care, and treatment patterns at different sites across one academic medical center. PLoS One 2019;14(7). https://doi.org/10.1371/journal.pone.0218388.
58. Miller JM, Binnicker MJ, Campbell S, et al. A guide to utilization of the microbiology laboratory for diagnosis of infectious diseases: 2018 update by the Infectious Diseases Society of America and the American Society for Microbiology. Clin Infect Dis 2018;67(6):e1–94.
59. Massachusetts Department of Public Health. 105 CMR 300: reportable diseases, surveillance, and isolation and quarantine requirements. Available at: https://www.mass.gov/regulations/105-CMR-30000-reportable-diseases-surveillance-and-isolation-and-quarantine. Accessed January 30, 2020.
60. Reller LB, Weinstein MP, Peterson LR, et al. Role of clinical microbiology laboratories in the management and control of infectious diseases and the delivery of health care. Clin Infect Dis 2001;32(4):605–10.

Infective Endocarditis in Persons Who Use Drugs
Epidemiology, Current Management, and Emerging Treatments

Asher Schranz, MD, MPH[a], Joshua A. Barocas, MD[b],*

KEYWORDS

• Infective endocarditis • Injection drug use • Substance use disorders • Opioids

KEY POINTS

- Infective endocarditis associated with injection drug use has increased substantially in North America.
- Infective endocarditis associated with injection drug use predominantly affects young persons and is primarily driven by *Staphylococcus aureus*.
- Infective endocarditis associated with injection drug use management involves antimicrobial therapy, heart valve surgery (if indicated), and evaluation for and treatment of coexisting substance use disorders.
- Although rates of in-hospital death are low in infective endocarditis associated with injection drug use, long-term outcomes are poor.

INTRODUCTION

Serious bacterial and fungal infections such as infective endocarditis (IE) are among the most common medical complications in persons who inject drugs (PWID).[1–3] IE once primarily impacted older adults and immunocompromised persons, but is increasingly common among younger persons as complications of injection drug use.[1,4–8] These infections can result in cardiac surgery,[9] sepsis, and death.[10,11] Herein, we review the epidemiology, current and emerging management strategies, clinical considerations and controversies, and propose an approach for the management of IE associated with injection drug use (IDU-IE).

[a] Division of Infectious Diseases, University of North Carolina-Chapel Hill, 130 Mason Farm Road (Bioinformatics), CB #7030, Chapel Hill, NC 27599-7030, USA; [b] Section of Infectious Diseases, Boston Medical Center, Boston University School of Medicine, 801 Massachusetts Avenue, 2nd Floor, Boston, MA 02118, USA
* Corresponding author.
E-mail address: Joshua.Barocas@bmc.org
Twitter: @asherjs (A.S.); @jabarocas (J.A.B.)

Infect Dis Clin N Am 34 (2020) 479–493
https://doi.org/10.1016/j.idc.2020.06.004
0891-5520/20/© 2020 Elsevier Inc. All rights reserved.

EPIDEMIOLOGY
Trends in Incidence and Mortality

In recent years, hospitalizations for IE have increased, driven by a surge in IDU-IE. In a nationally representative sample of US hospitalizations from 2000 to 2013, IE hospitalizations increased 38% overall, but hospitalizations for IDU-IE increased 238%.[7] More recent analyses of US population-based data have demonstrated continued uptrends in IDU-IE hospitalizations, with estimates as high as a 12-fold increase between 2007 and 2017.[9,12–14] Canada has also seen an upsurge in IDU-IE cases. In Ontario, rates of admissions more than doubled since the end of 2011.[15] The increase in IDU-IE is likely not consistent across regions in North America. In a comparison of 2 urban counties in Pennsylvania, Alleghany county experienced an increase in IDU-IE hospitalizations that was nearly 3-fold higher than Philadelphia, at 443% and 112%, respectively.[13] Of note, these large-scale, population-based analyses draw on administrative data and use billing codes for the identification of IDU-IE.

Numerous single- and multicenter studies have further characterized the increase in IDU-IE in greater clinical detail and confirmed that an increasing proportion of IE hospitalizations and surgeries are for IDU-IE. In a large hospital in North Carolina, IDU-IE increased to 56% of IE hospitalizations in 2014, from just 14% in 2009.[16] Furthermore, among patients who underwent heart valve surgery for IE across 8 academic centers in 2017, 28% were for IDU-IE, up from 19% in 2012,[8] echoing trends seen in other studies of IE surgeries.[9,17] Last, IDU-IE now accounts for increased mortality. In a study of US death certificates, there was a 3-fold increase in IDU-IE as a cause of death from 1999 to 2016, compared with an only 1.5-fold increase in IE deaths overall.[8]

Demographics

Persons with IDU-IE have a demographic and clinical profile that is, distinct from those with those with IE owing to other causes (non–IDU-IE). Most notably, patients with IDU-IE are consistently younger than patients with non–IDU-IE. In a nationally representative sample of patients with IDU-IE in the United States, the mean age was 38 years (vs 50 years for non–IDU-IE).[12] Persons with IDU-IE are also more commonly homeless (17%–21%)[11,18] and/or experience significant poverty.[14,15] Hepatitis C virus infection is frequent (36%–82%). Many studies report that 45% to 55% of patients with IDU-IE are female[9,13,15,19]; however, one study found that females accounted for only 13% of patients undergoing surgery.[20]

There remains substantial heterogeneity in the demographics of patients with IDU-IE by region, which likely reflects variation in the epidemiology of PWID. For example, although the majority of patients with IDU-IE in the United States are non-Hispanic and white, non-white patients comprised 40% of IDU-IE hospitalizations in the Northeast, but only 27% in the South.[14]

Clinical Characteristics

Although all 4 heart valves can be affected, IDU-IE most commonly involves the tricuspid valve (58%–77% of cases).[11,21,22] Surgical intervention most commonly occurs on the aortic valve (40%–64%), followed by the mitral valve (36%–45%) and the tricuspid valve (28%–39%), and many patients with IDU-IE undergo surgery on multiple valves (20%–54%).[9,13,23] The reasons for the predominance of left-sided valves in surgery is unclear, but may reflect infections with more embolic phenomena or poorer response to medical therapy than tricuspid disease.

IDU-IE results from bacteria entering the bloodstream from the skin or injection equipment, including syringes, needles, cookers, cottons, and water. As such, a variety of organisms are implicated in IDU-IE, including bacteria and fungi. Among bacteria, *Staphylococcus aureus* is the most common organism in IE, whether owing to drug use or not.[24] It is involved in 43% to 95% of first-episode IDU-IE and accounts for 20% to 63% of recurrent infections.[21–23] Unfortunately, a growing proportion of IDU-IE cases occur as the result of antimicrobial-resistant organisms. To date, many of these infections have included MRSA, which have more than doubled in recent years in this population.[25] Furthermore, although it affects only a small proportion of patients, fungal endovascular infections, specifically *Candida spp.,* merit special attention given their growing prevalence PWID and the challenges they pose to clinical management. In a large US surveillance study from 2017, 11% of patients with candidal bloodstream infections (candidemia) had a history of IDU, and the proportion of patients with candidemia who had injected drugs more than doubled from 2014 to 2017.[20] Fungal endocarditis is uncommon in first-time infections, but is more common in recurrent infections (7%–14%).[21,22]

Opioids are involved in a majority of reported IDU-IE cases, although there is variation by region. For example, in a cohort from Maine, heroin was the most common drug used by persons with IDU-IE and was associated with 60% of the infections.[18] In contrast, in a hospital in central North Carolina, prescription opioids were involved in 68% to 96% of IDU-IE.[21] Stimulants, such as cocaine and methamphetamine comprise substantial proportions in those studies (19%–31%). Current public health reports indicate increasing overdoses owing to both stimulants and combined stimulant/opioid use.[26,27] A series of IDU-associated infections in Western New York from 2017 found that a majority of patients use both cocaine and opioids (69%), although these patients primarily had skin and soft tissue infections and only 14% had IE.[28] As the epidemiology of the drug epidemic in North America continues to change, we expect fentanyl and other illicitly produced synthetic opioids, as well as stimulants, to be implicated in more IDU-IE cases. Future studies are needed to delineate the prevalence of these substances and polysubstance use in IDU-IE to inform the addiction care needs of this population.

DISCUSSION
Current Management Strategies

The management of IDU-IE is generally consistent with the management of non–IDU-IE, which may include medical or combined medical-surgical therapy. The care of persons with IDU-IE should also include components to address the underlying substance use disorder (SUD).

Medical management
Antimicrobial treatment for IE generally consists of 2 to 6 weeks of parenteral antibiotics. Antibiotic choice and duration are tailored based on the organism species and its antimicrobial susceptibility profile, the presence of a prosthetic valve or other material, the patient's ability to tolerate specific antimicrobials, and tissue penetration to areas of metastatic or distant infection. Full details of antimicrobial regimens are delineated in the guidelines published by the American Heart Association and endorsed by the Infectious Diseases Society of America, and are generally not unique for IDU-IE.[29] Although most antimicrobial courses are 4 to 6 weeks, a notable exception is short-course therapy for uncomplicated tricuspid endocarditis in IDU-IE owing to methicillin-susceptible *S aureus*, where an anti-Staphylococcal penicillin can be given intravenously for 2 weeks.[30,31]

Home intravenous antibiotics can be a safe option for select PWID that also decreases costs and hospital duration.[32–34] Observational cohort studies have shown that PWID (housed and homeless) can achieve good cure rates.[35] Fanucchi and colleagues[33] (2019) demonstrated the feasibility and effectiveness of outpatient parenteral antimicrobial therapy for PWID in a pilot randomized trial. In their model, they found that outpatient parenteral antimicrobial therapy provided in an integrated outpatient model that includes medications for opioid use disorder (MOUD) treatment for severe injection-related infection has clinical outcomes that are similar to those of prolonged hospitalization while shortening the hospital length of stay.

Surgical management

For patients with IE—drug related or otherwise—decisions about valve surgery must be individualized. Surgery before the completion of antibiotics (ie, "early" surgery) is most commonly considered on the basis of anatomic and structural concerns, such as new valvular regurgitation and symptomatic right or left heart failure or heart block, which may be a presenting sign of an intracardiac abscess.[29] Other reasons to consider early surgery include persistent bacteremia, ongoing embolic phenomena or large vegetations (>10 mm on the anterior leaflet of the mitral valve or ≥20 mm on the tricuspid valve). Finally, certain organisms, which are more common in IDU-IE, such as Pseudomonas aeruginosa and fungi, indicate early surgical consideration owing to their association with high mortality (>40% and >60%, respectively).[36–38]

Several studies support the role of surgery during the initial hospitalization for left-sided native valve IE.[39–41] Observational data on prosthetic valve IE have shown that patients with strong surgical indications also benefit from early surgery.[42] However, these studies have not specified IDU-IE within the population, except one, which included only 9 such cases.[40] Despite the association between surgery and improved outcomes, aortic valve surgeries for IE have decreased since 2013 for both IDU-IE and IE overall.[43]

There seems to be little rationale for systematically withholding surgery in PWID. In fact, surgical intervention for first-episode IDU-IE has been associated with improved all-cause mortality in 1 cohort of Canadian patients.[11] Surgery typically includes open valve replacement or repair, that latter of which is performed less commonly than replacement.[23] Valvectomy is an option for source control for tricuspid valve IE nonresponsive to medical therapy, although it is rarely performed. Although most surgeries address only 1 valve, 22% to 25% involve 2 valves and 3% to 4% target 3 vales. There is also accumulating evidence for the use of a vacuum-assisted percutaneous debridement of tricuspid vegetations in IDU-IE.[44,45] This device has been used in patients with hemodynamic compromise or other acute comorbidities felt to render them poor surgical candidates and has also been used as a strategy for source control. Although patient outcomes have generally been favorable in these case series, further data are needed to determine indications for using this approach.

Addiction management

IE among PWID is the result of an unaddressed SUD. If the underlying SUD remains untreated, patients are likely to experience poor outcomes. As such, MOUD—naltrexone, buprenorphine, and methadone—and addiction treatment should be considered essential components of treatment for IDU-IE. The National Academies of Medicine, Science and Engineering have specifically highlighted the need for inpatient OUD care as a key action step in addressing the intersection of the opioid epidemic and infectious diseases.[46]

Studies integrating IE and OUD treatment in both the inpatient and outpatient settings have shown promising results.[33,47–49] In a cohort of patients with IDU-IE from

Ontario, Canada, addiction treatment referral was the only factor aside from surgery that improved mortality.[11] In a study from Missouri, inpatient addiction consultation for patients with infections was strongly associated with antibiotic completion, fewer discharges against medical advice (AMA), and increased MOUD receipt.[50] MOUD receipt remains rare; less than 12% of patients with IDU-IE are discharged with a plan to start an MOUD.[51,52] Multidisciplinary IE treatment teams that provide a comprehensive inpatient treatment package are sensible interventions to coordinate care and improve patient outcomes. These teams may include cardiologists, cardiac surgeons, hospitalists, addiction medicine, and infectious diseases specialists, as well as case managers to help address underlying social and structural issues that are often barriers to retention in care and recovery.

Additionally, patients can benefit from harm reduction services. Harm reduction is an approach to care that aims to nonjudgmentally determine where a person is with respect to motivation for behavior change and to offer them care to improve their health, starting at that point.[53] Often applied in settings of substance use, harm reduction services can include those that focus on ensuring that patients have access to sterile injection equipment, that they are educated on safer injection practices (eg, cleaning skin, using sterile water, heating cookers), and that they receive naloxone and overdose education. The implementation of harm reduction education in the hospital or helping patients to link to syringe service programs at discharge may help to decrease the risk of repeat infections and fatal overdoses.

Clinical Outcomes

Short and long term

In the early period after IDU-IE, patients have relatively good outcomes. In-hospital mortality has been reported at 5% to 10% and is consistently lower than those hospitalized for IE owing to reasons other than injecting drugs.[9,12–14,18] For patients undergoing valve surgery for IDU-IE, in-hospital and 30-day mortality is no different between IDU-IE and non–IDU-IE.[54]

Long-term outcomes after IDU-IE are not as good and likely reflect the inadequate state of addiction care delivered to patients with IDU-IE. For those undergoing surgery, mortality seems to worsen, compared with those with non–IDU-IE, in the midterm postoperative period (eg, at the 3- or 6-month timepoints).[55,56] The 1-year mortality in North America has been reported to be 16% to 20%.[11,19] A cohort from Boston had a 26% mortality rate at a median of 306 days of follow-up, with a median age of death of 41 years, underscoring the devastating consequences of IDU-IE to young persons.[51] Although data on very long-term outcomes (>5 years) are limited, 1 meta-analysis reported 5- and 10-year postoperative mortality at a dismal 62% and 57%, respectively, with a higher hazard ratio for IDU-IE, compared with others with IE (hazard ratio, 1.47; 95% confidence interval, 1.05–2.05).[57]

One factor contributing to posthospitalization outcomes is the relatively high proportion of AMA discharges in IDU-IE. Of hospitalizations for IDU-IE, 5% to 22% result in AMA discharges, compared with 1% to 2% among other IE patients.[9,12,13,58] These discharges almost certainly indicate a truncation in care for a serious infection and implore providers to address the root causes of this outcome. AMA discharges are driven by numerous factors, including negative experiences with staff and inadequate pain management.[59] Given that SUDs are largely inadequately addressed and treated during a hospitalization,[51,60] patients may experience drug withdrawal syndromes contributing to their decision to leave the hospital.[59,61]

Clinical Considerations

Infectious diseases involvement in addiction care

Infectious diseases providers can play a unique role in the care of SUD in the context of IDU-IE and comparable invasive injection-related infections, such as spinal, bone, joint, and severe soft tissue infections, as well as typically chronic infections, such as human immunodeficiency virus and viral hepatitis. Encountered with such patients regularly, it is sensible for ID providers to undertake prescribing of MOUD and naloxone, provide education on safer injection practices, and refer patients to syringe service programs, where available.[62,63] Guidelines for the care of hepatitis C virus already specifically recommend that providers include MOUD, referral to syringe service programs, and overdose education alongside direct acting antivirals.[64] Persons with invasive injection-related infections would also greatly benefit from these resources.

Recurrent valve surgery

Recurrent IE is common among PWID and is associated with significant mortality. In a cohort of 87 PWID with IDU-IE, 25% experienced recurrent IE, the majority of which occurred within 1 year of the first episode.[21] Of those with recurrent IE, nearly one-quarter required surgical intervention and more than one-third died within 1 year. Within the medical and surgical communities, uncertainty remains regarding the initial and, more commonly, repeat valve surgery in IDU-IE. One qualitative study of health care providers showed a wide range of opinions on how to approach repeat valve surgeries, from those who recommended strict single surgery policies to those who felt patients should be offered as many surgeries as needed.[65] A bioethical analysis has highlighted that some of the opinions surrounding offering recurrent valve surgery may be informed by feelings of underpreparedness in treating IDU-IE, implicit and explicit bias, and a lack of transparency in criteria for surgical decision making. Clearly, a patient-centered approach and thoughtful guidance from a multidisciplinary group is necessary for optimal patient care.

Emerging Treatment Approaches

There are a number of emerging treatment approaches that hold the potential to redefine our approach to IDU-IE. First, few studies have assessed the efficacy of oral antibiotic regimens for IE. Two small trials have examined oral therapy for native valve IE and found satisfactory cure rates for oral therapy in right-sided IE in PWID, and in partial oral therapy for left-sided disease.[66] More recently, Iversen and colleagues (2018)[67] conducted a large randomized noninferiority, multicenter trial to determine if partial oral antibiotic treatment resulted in similar efficacy and safety as a full course of intravenous treatment. The Partial Oral Treatment of Endocarditis (POET) Trial randomized 400 patients with stable left-sided disease to either a full intravenous antibiotic course or a switch to an oral regimen after initial intravenous antibiotics. The composite outcome of the trial was all-cause mortality, unplanned cardiac surgery, embolic events, or relapse of bacteremia with the primary pathogen, from the time of randomization until 6 months after antibiotic treatment was completed. The composite outcome occurred in 12.1% in the intravenously treated group and in 9.0% in the orally treated group, resulting in a between-group difference of 3.1% points, which met noninferiority criteria. Although these results are promising for the population at large, there are reasons that these findings should be interpreted with caution in the setting of PWID. First, although the study did include patients with *S aureus* endocarditis (n = 35), none were identified as methicillin resistant. Conversely, invasive methicillin-resistant *S aureus* is among the commonest pathogens in endocarditis among PWID in North America[21,25]; therefore, findings from this trial may not be generalizable to patients with methicillin-resistant *S aureus* endocarditis. Second, there were only 5 PWID out of the 400 total enrollees in this trial (1.25%). There is, however, no reason to believe that oral antibiotics are less biologically effective in PWID than in those who do not inject drugs. Overall, the POET trial adds to an emerging evidence-base for oral antibiotics in the treatment of endocarditis and provides a launching pad for further research in IDU-IE.

Long-acting glycopeptides are also emerging as a potential treatment for endocarditis, although experience is limited. Dalbavancin and oritavancin have been approved by the US Food and Drug Administration for the treatment of acute skin and skin structure infections caused by gram-positive bacteria. They are administered intravenously, but their long half-lives allow for weekly dosing, making them appealing choices for persons requiring parenteral therapy for prolonged durations. Phase II studies for complicated bacteremia and endocarditis have ended, but data remain forthcoming. Retrospective observational cohorts and case series are emerging regarding their efficacy and safety. Tobudic and colleagues[68] performed a 2-year retrospective analysis of adults with endocarditis who were treated with dalbavancin. In this series of 27 patients with a mix of prosthetic and native valves, organisms, and therapies before dalbavancin, the authors noted that 93% of patients achieved microbiological and clinical success. Another retrospective series among people who use drugs with serious gram-positive infections demonstrated similar results. Bryson-Cahn and colleagues[69] noted that none of the 9 patients with endocarditis were known to have failed dalbavancin step-down treatment, but 4 (44%) were lost to follow-up. A number of other observational studies have corroborated these findings and suggest that dalbavancin may be effective as consolidation therapy in patients with endocarditis following initial treatment with approved intravenous antibiotics.[70–72] Evidence for the treatment of endocarditis with oritavancin is more scarce.[73]

In addition to uncertain efficacy, other barriers to treatment uptake with long-acting glycopeptides exist. First, some argue that the cost of these medications does not justify their use. Given that dalbavancin is not approved by the US Food and Drug Administration for endocarditis, insurers may decline to cover its cost, thereby shifting the cost to hospitals and patients. However, multiple analyses have suggested that costs to the system may be offset by decreased hospital length of stay.[72,74] Further research is needed to examine the economic impact and cost effectiveness of these antibiotics. Another barrier to dalbavancin use is the lack of a defined optimal dosing and monitoring schedules. Several dosing strategies have been proposed that include once and twice weekly dosing with variable loading and maintenance dosages.[68,69] Despite anecdotal success, more rigorous evaluation is clearly needed.

Barriers to Treating Endocarditis

A number of barriers have been discussed elsewhere in this article; however, we have identified 2 important system-level barriers to treating endocarditis in PWID: lack of infrastructure and work force and the rapidly evolving North American drug epidemic.

First, in a recent survey of infectious diseases physicians, only 22% reported that their primary hospital provided a dedicated multidisciplinary addiction service.[62] These respondents were significantly more likely to agree or strongly agree that physicians should actively manage SUDs than were physicians whose facilities did not provide a dedicated service. Furthermore, although nearly one-half of the respondents felt that infectious diseases providers should actively manage SUDs, only 3% reported having a waiver from the US Drug Enforcement Agency to prescribe buprenorphine in the outpatient setting. To overcome this barrier, more providers are needed who are willing and able to prescribe buprenorphine. Reevaluating restrictive federal policies, such as eliminating the requirement for a waiver to prescribe outpatient buprenor-phine,[75] would likely expand treatment access.[76] Additionally, a large proportion (34%–57%) of those hospitalized with injection-related infections in studies from states that did not expand Medicaid were uninsured,[9,34] limiting the availability of outpatient services and MOUD. Medicaid expansion has been linked to improved OUD-related outcomes such as overdose[77] and would conceivably also have a positive effect on IDU-IE outcomes.

Second, drug overdose data suggest that persons using drugs are shifting from using opioids only to polysubstance use that includes stimulants (ie, cocaine and meth-amphetamine). This evolution poses significant challenges to addressing IDU-IE, given that stimulant use disorder lacks effective pharmacotherapies, unlike OUD. With no approved treatments for stimulant use disorder, few addiction providers to

---

Box 1
Recommended components of inpatient care for persons with injection drug use-associated IE

IE care

Antimicrobial therapy
• Empiric therapy
• Narrowed, organism-directed therapy based on culture data[a]

Cardiac surgery consultation

Screening for viral infections impacting PWID
• See **Box 2**

Immunization for certain infections of concern in PWID
• See **Box 2**

Dental prophylaxis[79]
• Prescription for amoxicillin 2 g once to be taken 30 to 60 minutes before the procedure
  ○ Alternative options for penicillin-allergic patients and parenteral options are available
• Patient education

Referral for outpatient follow-up care with infectious diseases and, if indicated, cardiology and cardiac surgery

SUD care

• Addiction medicine consultation (where available)

• For support where no specialized addiction consultation is available, providers requesting clinical assistance should utilize peer mentoring through:
  ○ "Warm line" clinician-to-clinician phone consultation (eg, https://nccc.ucsf.edu/clinical-resources/substance-use-resources/)
  ○ Project ECHO (Extension for Community Healthcare Outcomes) sessions for opioid use disorder care (eg, https://echo.unc.edu/; https://www.bmcobat.org/project-echo/massachusetts-obat-echo/)
  ○ Direct mentoring from experienced clinicians (eg, https://pcssnow.org/mentoring/)

• Offer of inpatient MOUD, notably buprenorphine and methadone
  ○ Attention should be paid to medication interactions and pain management needs

• Referral to outpatient addiction treatment provider

• Naloxone prescription and overdose education

• Information for accessible syringe services program, where legal and available

[a] Full details of antimicrobial regimens are available in guidelines published by the American Heart Association.[29]

Box 2
Screening, immunization, and prophylaxis recommendations for infectious diseases in hospitalized PWID

Hepatitis A
- Screening for preexisting immunity: hepatitis A IgG
- Immunization: 2-dose vaccine; interval between doses depends on vaccine preparation

Hepatitis B
- Screening: surface antigen, core IgG, and surface antibody
- Immunization: if all of the above are negative, immunize with 2- or 3-dose vaccine series[a]

Hepatitis C
- Screening: hepatitis C antibody with reflex to RNA; for persons with known antibody positivity, screen with hepatitis C RNA

Tetanus
- Immunization
  - Adults without documented prior receipt of tetanus toxoid, reduced diphtheria toxoid, and acellular pertussis (Tdap) vaccine should receive 1 dose of Tdap
  - Adults with prior documented Tdap should receive a tetanus and diphtheria toxoids (Td) booster vaccine if 10 years have elapsed since their last documented tetanus and diphtheria vaccine

Pneumococcus
- Immunization: 1-time dose of 23-valent pneumococcal polysaccharide vaccine for patients with chronic heart, lung, or liver disease; alcohol use disorder; or cigarette smoking, as well as certain other chronic medical conditions, asplenia or immunocompromising conditions

Human immunodeficiency virus
- Preexposure prophylaxis can be offered to patients at risk of human immunodeficiency virus acquisition from injecting drugs or sex
- Postexposure prophylaxis can be offered to persons with high-risk exposure and as a bridge to preexposure prophylaxis[80]

Special situations exist for the immunization of pregnant women or those with incomplete or unknown vaccination or other special populations. Consult recommendations from the American Committee on Immunization Practices for full details.[a] The 2-dose, novel adjuvant hepatitis B vaccine is given across a 4-week interval and, thus, a full vaccination series may be possible during a hospitalization for patients who remain hospitalized for the full duration of IE therapy.

---

engage with patients, and areas with insufficient harm reduction infrastructure,[78] it is possible that increasing stimulant use will herald increases in IE and other invasive bacterial and fungal infections.

Proposed Treatment Recommendations

In the absence of comprehensive, multidisciplinary clinical guidelines, we propose the following treatment paradigm for IE among PWID in **Boxes 1** and **2**. We strongly encourage a standardized management approach to decrease variability owing to provider or institutional beliefs. In clinical settings where electronic health records exist, this can be facilitated by a standardized endocarditis order set.

SUMMARY

Endocarditis among PWID is an increasingly common problem associated with significant morbidity and mortality. Much like increasing hepatitis C virus infections and mounting outbreaks of human immunodeficiency virus, endocarditis has increased alongside the US drug epidemic. Addressing SUD is a key element of comprehensive care, and more work is need to integrate efforts to address endocarditis treatment, the underlying SUD and structural factors that might limit retention in care, long-term recovery, and prevention of infections. There remains an urgent need for multidisciplinary guidelines and best practices that are tailored to the unique needs of people who use drugs with endocarditis.

CLINICS CARE POINTS

- Patients with IE and opioid use disorder should be offered MOUD during the hospitalization or perihospitalization period.
- Outpatient parenteral antibiotic treatment can be considered in the treatment of IDU-IE for certain patients. Future management strategies may include oral antibiotics and long-acting glycopeptides.
- Discussions regarding co-occurring SUDs, injection practices, and overdose risk should take place with all patients with injection-related endocarditis.
- All patients should be counseled regarding the principles of harm reduction, including safer injection practices, and be provided with overdose education and naloxone upon hospital discharge.

DISCLOSURE

Dr J.A. Barocas reports receiving funding from the Charles A. King Trust and from the National Institute on Drug Abuse (R01DA046527-02S1).

REFERENCES

1. Ciccarone D, Unick GJ, Cohen JK, et al. Nationwide increase in hospitalizations for heroin-related soft tissue infections: associations with structural market conditions. Drug Alcohol Depend 2016;163:126–33.

2. Larney S, Peacock A, Mathers BM, et al. A systematic review of injecting-related injury and disease among people who inject drugs. Drug Alcohol Depend 2017; 171:39–49.

3. Dwyer R, Topp L, Maher L, et al. Prevalences and correlates of non-viral injecting-related injuries and diseases in a convenience sample of Australian injecting drug users. Drug Alcohol Depend 2009;100(1–2):9–16.

4. Fleischauer AT, Ruhl L, Rhea S, et al. Hospitalizations for endocarditis and associated health care costs among persons with diagnosed drug dependence - North Carolina, 2010-2015. MMWR Morb Mortal Wkly Rep 2017;66(22):569–73.

5. Miller AC, Polgreen PM. Many opportunities to record, diagnose, or treat injection drug-related infections are missed: a population-based cohort study of inpatient and emergency department settings. Clin Infect Dis 2019;68(7):1166–75.

6. Gray ME, Rogawski McQuade ET, Scheld WM, et al. Rising rates of injection drug use associated infective endocarditis in Virginia with missed opportunities for addiction treatment referral: a retrospective cohort study. BMC Infect Dis 2018; 18(1):532.

7. Wurcel AG, Anderson JE, Chui KK, et al. Increasing infectious endocarditis admissions among young people who inject drugs. Open Forum Infect Dis 2016; 3(3):ofw157.

8. Njoroge LW, Al-Kindi SG, Koromia GA, et al. Changes in the association of rising infective endocarditis with mortality in people who inject drugs. JAMA Cardiol 2018;3(8):779–80.
9. Schranz AJ, Fleischauer A, Chu VH, et al. Trends in drug use-associated infective endocarditis and heart valve surgery, 2007 to 2017: a study of statewide discharge data. Ann Intern Med 2019;170(1):31–40.
10. Straw S, Baig MW, Gillott R, et al. Long-term outcomes are poor in intravenous drug users following infective endocarditis, even after surgery. Clin Infect Dis 2019. [Epub ahead of print].
11. Rodger L, Glockler-Lauf SD, Shojaei E, et al. Clinical characteristics and factors associated with mortality in first-episode infective endocarditis among persons who inject drugs. JAMA Netw Open 2018;1(7):e185220.
12. Rudasill SE, Sanaiha Y, Mardock AL, et al. Clinical outcomes of infective endocarditis in injection drug users. J Am Coll Cardiol 2019;73(5):559–70.
13. Meisner JA, Anesi J, Chen X, et al. Changes in infective endocarditis admissions in Pennsylvania during the opioid epidemic. Clin Infect Dis 2019. [Epub ahead of print].
14. Kadri AN, Wilner B, Hernandez AV, et al. Geographic trends, patient characteristics, and outcomes of infective endocarditis associated with drug abuse in the United States from 2002 to 2016. J Am Heart Assoc 2019;8(19):e012969.
15. Weir MA, Slater J, Jandoc R, et al. The risk of infective endocarditis among people who inject drugs: a retrospective, population-based time series analysis. CMAJ 2019;191(4):E93–9.
16. Hartman L, Barnes E, Bachmann L, et al. Opiate injection-associated infective endocarditis in the Southeastern United States. Am J Med Sci 2016;352(6):603–8.
17. Kim JB, Ejiofor JI, Yammine M, et al. Surgical outcomes of infective endocarditis among intravenous drug users. J Thorac Cardiovasc Surg 2016;152(3): 832–41.e1.
18. Thakarar K, Rokas KE, Lucas FL, et al. Mortality, morbidity, and cardiac surgery in Injection Drug Use (IDU)-associated versus non-IDU infective endocarditis: the need to expand substance use disorder treatment and harm reduction services. PLoS One 2019;14(11):e0225460.
19. Leahey PA, LaSalvia MT, Rosenthal ES, et al. High morbidity and mortality among patients with sentinel admission for injection drug use-related infective endocarditis. Open Forum Infect Dis 2019;6(4):ofz089.
20. Nguemeni Tiako MJ, Mori M, Bin Mahmood SU, et al. Recidivism is the leading cause of death among intravenous drug users who underwent cardiac surgery for infective endocarditis. Semin Thorac Cardiovasc Surg 2019;31(1):40–5.
21. Huang G, Barnes EW, Peacock JE Jr. Repeat infective endocarditis in persons who inject drugs: "take another little piece of my heart. Open Forum Infect Dis 2018;5(12):ofy304.
22. Rodger L, Shah M, Shojaei E, et al. Recurrent endocarditis in persons who inject drugs. Open Forum Infect Dis 2019;6(10):ofz396.
23. Mori M, Bin Mahmood SU, Schranz AJ, et al. Risk of reoperative valve surgery for endocarditis associated with drug use. J Thorac Cardiovasc Surg 2020;159(4): 1262–8.e2.
24. Murdoch DR, Corey GR, Hoen B, et al. Clinical presentation, etiology, and outcome of infective endocarditis in the 21st century: the International Collaboration on Endocarditis-Prospective Cohort Study. Arch Intern Med 2009;169(5): 463–73.

25. Jackson KA, Bohm MK, Brooks JT, et al. Invasive methicillin-resistant staphylococcus aureus infections among persons who inject drugs - six sites, 2005-2016. MMWR Morb Mortal Wkly Rep 2018;67(22):625–8.

26. Kariisa M, Scholl L, Wilson N, et al. Drug overdose deaths involving cocaine and psychostimulants with abuse potential - United States, 2003-2017. MMWR Morb Mortal Wkly Rep 2019;68(17):388–95.

27. Seth P, Scholl L, Rudd RA, et al. Overdose deaths involving opioids, cocaine, and psychostimulants - United States, 2015-2016. MMWR Morb Mortal Wkly Rep 2018;67(12):349–58.

28. Hartnett KP, Jackson KA, Felsen C, et al. Bacterial and fungal infections in persons who inject drugs - Western New York, 2017. MMWR Morb Mortal Wkly Rep 2019;68(26):583–6.

29. Baddour LM, Wilson WR, Bayer AS, et al. Infective endocarditis in adults: diagnosis, antimicrobial therapy, and management of complications: a scientific statement for healthcare professionals from the American Heart Association. Circulation 2015;132(15):1435–86.

30. Ribera E, Gomez-Jimenez J, Cortes E, et al. Effectiveness of cloxacillin with and without gentamicin in short-term therapy for right-sided Staphylococcus aureus endocarditis. A randomized, controlled trial. Ann Intern Med 1996;125(12):969–74.

31. Fortun J, Navas E, Martinez-Beltran J, et al. Short-course therapy for right-side endocarditis due to Staphylococcus aureus in drug abusers: cloxacillin versus glycopeptides in combination with gentamicin. Clin Infect Dis 2001;33(1):120–5.

32. D'Couto HT, Robbins GK, Ard KL, et al. Outcomes according to discharge location for persons who inject drugs receiving outpatient parenteral antimicrobial therapy. Open Forum Infect Dis 2018;5(5):ofy056.

33. Fanucchi LC, Walsh SL, Thornton AC, et al. Outpatient parenteral antimicrobial therapy plus buprenorphine for opioid use disorder and severe injection-related infections. Clin Infect Dis 2020;70(6):1226–9.

34. Eaton EF, Mathews RE, Lane PS, et al. A 9-point risk assessment for patients who inject drugs and require intravenous antibiotics: focusing inpatient resources on patients at greatest risk of ongoing drug use. Clin Infect Dis 2019;68(6):1041–3.

35. Suzuki J, Johnson J, Montgomery M, et al. Outpatient parenteral antimicrobial therapy among people who inject drugs: a review of the literature. Open Forum Infect Dis 2018;5(9):ofy194.

36. Pierrotti LC, Baddour LM. Fungal endocarditis, 1995-2000. Chest 2002;122(1):302–10.

37. Cohen PS, Maguire JH, Weinstein L. Infective endocarditis caused by gram-negative bacteria: a review of the literature, 1945-1977. Prog Cardiovasc Dis 1980;22(4):205–42.

38. Arnold CJ, Johnson M, Bayer AS, et al. Candida infective endocarditis: an observational cohort study with a focus on therapy. Antimicrob Agents Chemother 2015;59(4):2365–73.

39. Lalani T, Cabell CH, Benjamin DK, et al. Analysis of the impact of early surgery on in-hospital mortality of native valve endocarditis: use of propensity score and instrumental variable methods to adjust for treatment-selection bias. Circulation 2010;121(8):1005–13.

40. Bannay A, Hoen B, Duval X, et al. The impact of valve surgery on short- and long-term mortality in left-sided infective endocarditis: do differences in methodological approaches explain previous conflicting results? Eur Heart J 2011;32(16):2003–15.

41. Kang DH, Lee S, Kim YJ, et al. Long-term results of early surgery versus conventional treatment for infective endocarditis trial. Korean Circ J 2016;46(6):846–50.

42. Lalani T, Chu VH, Park LP, et al. In-hospital and 1-year mortality in patients undergoing early surgery for prosthetic valve endocarditis. JAMA Intern Med 2013; 173(16):1495–504.

43. Kimmel SD, Walley AY, Linas BP, et al. Effect of publicly reported aortic valve surgery outcomes on valve surgery in injection drug- and non-injection drug-associated endocarditis. Clin Infect Dis 2019. [Epub ahead of print].

44. George B, Voelkel A, Kotter J, et al. A novel approach to percutaneous removal of large tricuspid valve vegetations using suction filtration and veno-venous bypass: a single center experience. Catheter Cardiovasc Interv 2017;90(6):1009–15.

45. Abubakar H, Rashed A, Subahi A, et al. AngioVac system used for vegetation debulking in a patient with tricuspid valve endocarditis: a case report and review of the literature. Case Rep Cardiol 2017;2017:1923505.

46. Springer SA, Korthuis PT, Del Rio C. Integrating treatment at the intersection of opioid use disorder and infectious disease epidemics in medical settings: a call for action after a National Academies of Sciences, Engineering, and Medicine Workshop. Ann Intern Med 2018;169(5):335–6.

47. Fanucchi LC, Walsh SL, Thornton AC, et al. Integrated outpatient treatment of opioid use disorder and injection-related infections: a description of a new care model. Prev Med 2019;128:105760.

48. Suzuki J. Medication-assisted treatment for hospitalized patients with intravenous-drug-use related infective endocarditis. Am J Addict 2016;25(3): 191–4.

49. Suzuki J, Johnson JA, Montgomery MW, et al. Long-term outcomes of injection drug-related infective endocarditis among people who inject drugs. J Addict Med 2019. [Epub ahead of print].

50. Marks LR, Munigala S, Warren DK, et al. Addiction medicine consultations reduce readmission rates for patients with serious infections from opioid use disorder. Clin Infect Dis 2019;68(11):1935–7.

51. Rosenthal ES, Karchmer AW, Theisen-Toupal J, et al. Suboptimal addiction interventions for patients hospitalized with injection drug use-associated infective endocarditis. Am J Med 2016;129(5):481–5.

52. Barocas JA, Morgan JR, Wang J, et al. Outcomes associated with medications for opioid use disorder among persons hospitalized for infective endocarditis. Clin Infect Dis 2020. [Epub ahead of print].

53. Logan DE, Marlatt GA. Harm reduction therapy: a practice-friendly review of research. J Clin Psychol 2010;66(2):201–14.

54. Hall R, Shaughnessy M, Boll G, et al. Drug use and postoperative mortality following valve surgery for infective endocarditis: a systematic review and meta-analysis. Clin Infect Dis 2019;69(7):1120–9.

55. Shrestha NK, Jue J, Hussain ST, et al. Injection drug use and outcomes after surgical intervention for infective endocarditis. Ann Thorac Surg 2015;100(3): 875–82.

56. Wurcel AG, Boll G, Burke D, et al. Impact of substance use disorder on midterm mortality after valve surgery for endocarditis. Ann Thorac Surg 2020;109(5): 1426–32.

57. Goodman-Meza D, Weiss RE, Gamboa S, et al. Long term surgical outcomes for infective endocarditis in people who inject drugs: a systematic review and meta-analysis. BMC Infect Dis 2019;19(1):918.

58. Schranz AJ, Wu LT, Wohl DA, et al. Readmission after discharge against medical advice for persons with opioid-associated infective endocarditis. Philadeplphia: American Health Association Scientific Sessions; 2019. p. 2019.
59. Simon R, Snow R, Wakeman S. Understanding why patients with substance use disorders leave the hospital against medical advice: a qualitative study. Subst Abus 2019. [Epub ahead of print].
60. Serota DP, Niehaus ED, Schechter MC, et al. Disparity in quality of infectious disease vs addiction care among patients with injection drug use-associated Staphylococcus aureus Bacteremia. Open Forum Infect Dis 2019;6(7):ofz289.
61. Bearnot B, Mitton JA, Hayden M, et al. Experiences of care among individuals with opioid use disorder-associated endocarditis and their healthcare providers: results from a qualitative study. J Subst Abuse Treat 2019;102:16–22.
62. Rapoport AB, Fischer LS, Santibanez S, et al. Infectious diseases physicians' perspectives regarding injection drug use and related infections, United States, 2017. Open Forum Infect Dis 2018;5(7):ofy132.
63. Serota DP, Barocas JA, Springer SA. Infectious complications of addiction: a call for a new subspecialty within infectious diseases. Clin Infect Dis 2020;70(5): 968–72.
64. AASLD-IDSA. Key Populations: identification and management of HCV in people who inject drugs. Recommendations for testing, managing, and treating hepatitis C. Available at: https://www.hcvguidelines.org/unique-populations/pwid. Accessed July 5, 2020.
65. Hayden M, Moore A. Attitudes and approaches towards repeat valve surgery in recurrent injection drug use-associated infective endocarditis: a qualitative study. J Addict Med 2020;14(3):217–23.
66. Al-Omari A, Cameron DW, Lee C, et al. Oral antibiotic therapy for the treatment of infective endocarditis: a systematic review. BMC Infect Dis 2014;14:140.
67. Iversen K, Ihlemann N, Gill SU, et al. Partial oral versus intravenous antibiotic treatment of endocarditis. N Engl J Med 2019;380(5):415–24.
68. Tobudic S, Forstner C, Burgmann H, et al. Dalbavancin as primary and sequential treatment for gram-positive infective endocarditis: 2-year experience at the General Hospital of Vienna. Clin Infect Dis 2018;67(5):795–8.
69. Bryson-Cahn C, Beieler AM, Chan JD, et al. Dalbavancin as secondary therapy for serious Staphylococcus aureus infections in a vulnerable patient population. Open Forum Infect Dis 2019;6(2):ofz028.
70. Dinh A, Duran C, Pavese P, et al. French national cohort of first use of dalbavancin: a high proportion of off-label use. Int J Antimicrob Agents 2019;54(5):668–72.
71. Kussmann M, Karer M, Obermueller M, et al. Emergence of a dalbavancin induced glycopeptide/lipoglycopeptide non-susceptible Staphylococcus aureus during treatment of a cardiac device-related endocarditis. Emerg Microbes Infect 2018;7(1):202.
72. Hidalgo-Tenorio C, Vinuesa D, Plata A, et al. DALBACEN cohort: dalbavancin as consolidation therapy in patients with endocarditis and/or bloodstream infection produced by gram-positive cocci. Ann Clin Microbiol Antimicrob 2019;18(1):30.
73. Stewart CL, Turner MS, Frens JJ, et al. Real-world experience with oritavancin therapy in invasive gram-positive infections. Infect Dis Ther 2017;6(2):277–89.
74. Wilke M, Worf K, Preisendorfer B, et al. Potential savings through single-dose intravenous Dalbavancin in long-term MRSA infection treatment - a health economic analysis using German DRG data. GMS Infect Dis 2019;7:Doc03.
75. SAMHSA. MAT statutes, regulations, and guidelines. Rockville (MD): Substance Abuse and Mental Health Services Administration; 2015.

76. Fatseas M, Auriacombe M. Why buprenorphine is so successful in treating opiate addiction in France. Curr Psychiatry Rep 2007;9(5):358–64.
77. Kravitz-Wirtz N, Davis CS, Ponicki WR, et al. Association of Medicaid expansion with opioid overdose mortality in the United States. JAMA Netw Open 2020;3(1): e1919066.
78. Kishore S, Hayden M, Rich J. Lessons from Scott County - progress or paralysis on harm reduction? N Engl J Med 2019;380(21):1988–90.
79. Wilson W, Taubert KA, Gewitz M, et al. Prevention of infective endocarditis: guidelines from the American Heart Association: a guideline from the American Heart Association Rheumatic Fever, Endocarditis, and Kawasaki Disease Committee, Council on Cardiovascular Disease in the Young, and the Council on Clinical Cardiology, Council on Cardiovascular Surgery and Anesthesia, and the Quality of Care and Outcomes Research Interdisciplinary Working Group. Circulation 2007;116(15):1736–54.
80. Taylor JL, Walley AY, Bazzi AR. Stuck in the window with you: HIV exposure prophylaxis in the highest risk people who inject drugs. Subst Abus 2019;40(4): 441–3.

Soft Tissue, Bone, and Joint Infections in People Who Inject Drugs

Carlos S. Saldana, MD[a,1], Darshali A. Vyas, MD[b,1],
Alysse G. Wurcel, MD, MS[c,*]

KEYWORDS

- Injection drug use • People who inject drugs • Infection
- Skin and soft tissue infection, cellulitis, abscess
- Bone and joint infection, arthritis, osteomyelitis • Harm reduction

KEY POINTS

- Skin manifestations of injection drug use can be infectious and noninfectious; a thorough and nonjudgmental history and physical examination are necessary.
- Whereas joint infections may present with overt signs, bone infections may present indolently and require a high index of suspicion.
- Clinicians should be comfortable discussing injection practices with patients in order to provide harm reduction counseling.
- Encounters with people who inject drugs for treatment of infections are also opportunities to engage in discussions about treatment of substance use disorder and preexposure prophylaxis for human immunodeficiency virus.

INTRODUCTION

Skin and soft tissue infections (SSTI) along with bone and joint infections represent a significant source of morbidity and mortality among people who inject drugs (PWID). Nationally, hospitalizations because of these infections have increased dramatically in recent years.[1,2] Several studies have identified SSTIs as the primary reason that PWID engage with the health care system.[3,4] When left untreated or inadequately treated, SSTI and bone and joint infection put PWID at high risk of worsening infections, amputations, and death.[5,6] This review aims to characterize risks, pathogenesis, and

Funding: 1KL2TR002545-01 (A.G. Wurcel).
[a] Division of Infectious Diseases, Emory University School of Medicine, Atlanta, Georgia, USA;
[b] Department of Medicine, Massachusetts General Hospital, 55 Fruit Street, Boston, MA 02114, USA; [c] Department of Medicine, Division of Geographic Medicine and Infectious Diseases, Tufts Medical Center, 800 Washington Street, Boston, MA 02111, USA
[1] Co-first authors.
* Corresponding author. 800 Washington Avenue, Boston, MA 02111.
E-mail address: awurcel@tuftsmedicalcenter.org

management of SSTI and bone and joint infection in PWID and review harm reduction tools that clinicians can use when counseling patients.

RISK FACTORS AND PATHOGENESIS

The development of localized SSTI in PWID is driven by the introduction of pathogens into the skin.[7] Bacteria may originate on the skin surface, from the introduction of contaminated drugs, or from injection equipment, such as syringes and related paraphernalia. Foreign bodies and substances in the skin and surrounding tissue can delay local immune response by impairing blood and lymphatic drainage, further predisposing to localized infections at the site of injection.[8,9] Infection can also occur from the injection of drugs used as cutting or diluting agents (eg, lidocaine, quinine, talc, mannitol) or contaminants introduced during manufacturing or storage (eg, soil, dust, bacterial spores).[10,11]

As the opioid epidemic continues, notable shifts in drug supply and injection practices merit attention for their ability to alter disease risks. In the 1970s, there were increases in infections related to black tar heroin—a relatively impure form of heroin produced in Mexico and primarily sold west of the Mississippi River. Black tar heroin is thicker, can require caustic diluents, and may be contaminated with bacterial spores leading to tetanus and botulism outbreaks.[12–14] About 40 years later, the introduction of fentanyl marked an important change in the epidemiology of injection drug use and infectious diseases in the United States.[15] As a likely consequence of its rapid onset and short duration, fentanyl has been associated with high-frequency injection and syringe-sharing practices that can place individuals at greater infection risk.[16–18] Recently, there is increasing evidence that specific formulation of opioids, including controlled-release oral opioids, supports survival of *Staphylococcus aureus* in injection equipment[19] and increases the risk of endocarditis in PWID.[20]

More recently, coinjection of stimulants with opioids[21,22] has increased. Although higher rates of SSTI have been reported among people who inject primarily heroin compared with cocaine or methamphetamine, this may be in part due to vulnerable socioeconomic conditions and more severe substance use disorder among the demographic of people who use heroin compared with those who use cocaine.[23] More recently, infection with viral hepatitis and human immunodeficiency virus (HIV) as well as SSTI, has been linked to injections of stimulants alone, as well as injection of stimulants and heroin or fentanyl simultaneously.[24–28] One explanation is that cocaine causes increased vasoconstriction and can predispose to tissue necrosis and a delayed immune system response at the site of infection.[29] There is also evidence that methamphetamines may directly impair the immune response to infection and induce *S aureus* biofilm production.[30]

CLINICAL PRESENTATION
Skin and Soft Tissue Infections

The diagnosis of cellulitis is made clinically after obtaining a history and physical examination.[7] SSTI often occurs at the site of injection. Although the antecubital fossa is a common place for injection, PWID may use veins throughout the body, including in the legs, feet, groin, or neck,[31] so a full physical examination should be completed. Beyond cellulitis, PWID are at risk for a spectrum of SSTI ranging from abscesses to thrombophlebitis and necrotizing fasciitis. Necrotizing ulcers may develop as a consequence of "skin popping," toxicity, and the irritant properties of the drug and adulterants.[32,33] Chronic venous insufficiency has been reported in up to 86% of PWID and can be related to frequent vein trauma, thrombosis, or blockage, or the lymphatic

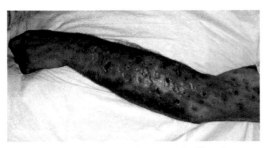

Fig. 1. Sclerosis and ulcers. (Image courtesy of Dr. David Effron.)

system.[34] Intraarterial injections occur when injecting vasoconstrictive agents directly into an artery, causing severe tissue ischemia and necrosis[35] and may mimic Raynaud phenomenon.[36] False aneurysms and mycotic aneurysms are rare but serious and are caused by vascular injuries after drug injection.[37]

Noninfectious dermatologic presentations should also be considered in PWID. Cutaneous nodules, panniculitis, sclerosis, and ulcers (**Fig. 1**) caused by dermal reactions to the drug and adulterants are frequently seen among PWID.[38,39] Hyperpigmentation and scarring (**Fig. 2**) are the most common cutaneous findings[40] related to various skin injuries. Cocaine has also been reported to cause a range of noninfectious dermatologic conditions, including Churg-Strauss vasculitis, Buerger disease, and scleroderma.[41] Notably, a rare complication of marijuana use is local arteritis, which most commonly affects the lower limbs and may present as Raynaud phenomenon or as claudication followed by the development of ulcers or gangrene, resembling Buerger disease.[42] Some adulterants may cause specific skin findings. Desomorphine, also known as "krokodil," can cause tissue damage as a result of contamination with substances used in the preparation of the drug. It leaves a green scaly appearance in the skin after injection, often accompanied by ulceration, which can become gangrenous (**Fig. 3**) and lead to sloughing of tissue down to the bone that often requires amputation.[43] Levamisole, another increasingly common adulterant detected in cocaine in the United States and worldwide,[44] may lead to a range of dermatologic manifestations, including lichen planus, erythema nodosum leprosum, nonspecific maculopapular rashes, and hemorrhagic bullae with a predilection for the ears and cheeks, and often has positive autoantibodies (eg, Anti-neutrophil cytoplasmic autoantibody [ANCA]).[45]

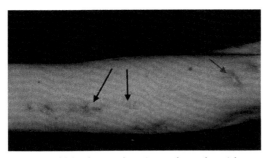

Fig. 2. Linear hyperpigmented bluish-gray heroin track marks with surrounding brown hyperpigmentation (*black arrows*), and leukodermic, depressed scar on the antecubital fossa, representing an area of frequent injection (*blue arrow*). (*From* Kazlouskaya, V., et al., A case of heroin linear track hyperpigmentation: histopathology and treatment with Q-switched Nd:YAG 1064nm laser. Int J Dermatol, 2018. 57(3): p. 362-364; with permission.)

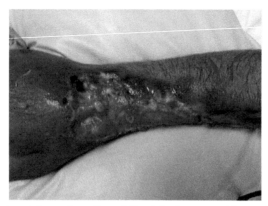

Fig. 3. Krokodil-induced deep ulceration of the right forearm with nearly exposed tendon. (*From* Haskin A et al, JAAD Case Rep. 2016 Mar; 2(2): 174–176; with permission.)

Bone and Joint Infections

Bone and joint infections generally result from hematogenous seeding or local extension of SSTIs. Any joint can be infected, although previous studies have found the knee and hip most commonly involved in PWID.[46] Septic tenosynovitis of distal extremities[47] and septic bursitis—most commonly in the olecranon and subdeltoid bursae—can occur.[48] Osteomyelitis can involve the extremities and appendicular skeleton in addition to the axial vertebrae—some studies have even reported a predominance of bone infections occurring in the extremities; however, most reports the location of bone and joint infection come from studies 20 to 30 years ago, and contemporary data are needed.[49–51]

Whereas SSTIs and septic arthritis often present with visible and/or systemic signs of infection like fever, osteomyelitis may present with only localized pain.[52] If the patient's pain is not taken seriously on presentation or if the patient is considered "drug-seeking,"[53] then the diagnosis may be delayed or missed. Untreated osteomyelitis can result in severe bone degradation, loss of function, fracture, and neurologic compromise,[54] rendering it a significant source of potential morbidity and mortality among PWID.[53]

MICROBIOLOGY

A wide range of organisms has been isolated in SSTIs and bone and joint infections. Up to 40% of SSTIs are polymicrobial.[55] Gram-positive cocci are most commonly identified.[56,57] Traditionally, injection drug use has been considered a risk factor for methicillin-resistant S aureus (MRSA) but according to more recent data,[55] S aureus (including MRSA)[58,59] is isolated less frequently among SSTIs in PWID compared with people who did not inject drugs. Common commensal organisms of the oral cavity, including *Streptococcus anginosus*, other viridans group streptococci, and anaerobic organisms are also identified in PWID and can thereby decrease the proportion of infections owing to MRSA.[55,60]

Similarly, up to 30% of bone and joint infections are polymicrobial.[56] The prevalence of Gram positives, including S aureus, *Staphylococcus epidermidis*, is the highest among PWID with bone and joint infections.[46] However, a high rate of infections with gram-negative organisms, especially *Pseudomonas aeruginosa* and other gram-negative bacilli and anaerobes, can also occur.[50] In addition, a higher rate of fungal infections occurs, including at unusual locations, such as the sternoclavicular joint.[61]

MANAGEMENT

Antimicrobial activity against both MRSA and streptococci is recommended for PWID until culture and susceptibilities become available. Recent evidence has shown that polymicrobial infections are also frequent in people who inject drugs, and broad-spectrum antibiotics should be considered.[55,62] Gram stains and cultures should be collected from pus drained directly from abscesses, if present. The decision to administer antibiotics as an adjunct to incision and drainage should be made based on the presence or absence of systemic symptoms. For deeper infections (necrotizing fasciitis, pyomyositis, myonecrosis, and so forth), surgical intervention is the primary therapeutic modality, and surgical consultation should be obtained when these infections are suspected.[62] Because examination alone might not be enough to rule out the presence of an abscess, especially for smaller or deeper collections, ultrasound should be considered to rule out abscess, which may require drainage for source control.[63]

Blood cultures have been found to be of low yield in SSTIs management. Current Infectious Diseases Society of America guidelines recommend against routine blood cultures in patients with SSTI, but still suggest that they may be indicated in PWID and in patients with fever.[62] A recent study[64] found that blood cultures had low yields of organisms in febrile patients and in PWID and were not significantly different than the yields in afebrile patients who do not inject drugs patients. Furthermore, all organisms from the blood cultures were susceptible to standard, empiric SSTI antibiotics, with little impact on patient management.[65]

There is limited consensus on empiric management of bone and joint infections in PWID. MRSA coverage with Vancomycin[56] plus a third- or fourth-generation cephalosporin[66] is a generally recommended empiric therapeutic option while awaiting definitive culture results. Empiric coverage for *Pseudomonas* and anaerobes (*Bacteroides fragilis* group, *Fusobacterium* spp, *Peptostreptococcus* spp, and *Propionibacterium acnes*)[67] should also be considered based on high-risk injection practices and local antibiogram.[46,56] To aid in the diagnosis of bone and joint infections (not SSTIs), blood cultures and inflammatory markers should be obtained in addition to basic laboratory studies. Elevated erythrocyte sedimentation rate/C-reactive protein levels are the most common laboratory abnormality found in the diagnosis of osteomyelitis, whereas other findings, such as leukocytosis, may or may not be present. Given the frequency of hematogenous spread, a set of blood cultures should always be sent before initiating empiric antibiotics in an attempt to isolate the causative organism. For septic arthritis, consultation with orthopedic surgery is essential, and joint fluid drainage should be performed.[66] It is important to monitor patients with septic arthritis closely with a low threshold to reaspirate a knee in the postoperative period and consider return to the operating room for more aggressive management.

Bone and joint infections typically require a prolonged antibiotic course. Some health care providers are reluctant to use peripherally inserted central catheters (PICC) in PWID.[68] A growing body of evidence has shown that outpatient parenteral antimicrobial therapy (OPAT) with a PICC line can be safe and effective for PWID, with rates of OPAT completion, mortality, and catheter-related complications comparable to those among people who do not inject drugs.[69] Providers should take into consideration patient preference and an individualized risk/benefit assessment.[70] The psychosocial risk assessment tool: "*Intravenous Antibiotics and Addiction Team (IVAT) 9-Point Risk Assessment*" can be used to help identify patients who may be able to complete outpatient antibiotics treatment.[71] Furthermore, innovative models that combine OPAT with buprenorphine treatment had similar clinical and drug use outcomes to usual care and significantly shortened length of stay.[72]

Notably, there is increasing data for alternatives to extended courses of intravenous (IV) antibiotics. The Oral versus Intravenous Antibiotics for Bone and Joint Infection Trial[73] demonstrated noninferiority of oral antibiotics compared with IV therapy in the management of these infections. Newer antibiotic formulations, such as Oritavancin (single-dose IV), Dalbavancin (single-dose IV), and Delafloxacin (IV/orally [PO]), have been studied in PWID and shown to expedite discharge in patients hospitalized with SSTIs.[74–76] Other agents, such as Omadacycline (IV/PO) and Tedizolid (IV/PO), are also promising and should be studied with prospective trials in this patient population.[77]

INCORPORATING HARM REDUCTION TOOLS

The provider should also be aware that the PWID may be hesitant to seek formal medical care when infectious complications develop given previous negative experiences with the health care system, and often instead resort to self-care.[78] PWID report inadequately treated pain, fear of precipitating acute withdrawal, and significant experiences with stigma and bias when seeking medical attention for infectious complications.[79] In a recent study, about one-third of PWID with a prior SSTI reported self-treating their infections to avoid or delay presenting to medical care by using methods, such as mechanical drainage, use of warm compress, and cleaning the area with alcohol/peroxide.[78,80] Reasons for delaying or avoiding medical attention for these infections vary and include not thinking the infections are severe, dislike or fear of the medical establishment, and fear of stigma.[80]

Given these experiences, adopting a harm reduction approach becomes critical for providers when caring for PWID. As used here, harm reduction refers to "a set of practical strategies and ideas aimed at reducing the negative consequences associated with drug use...built on a belief in, and respect for, the rights of people who use drugs."[81] Importantly, this approach comes without the expectation of abstinence from substances. With the understanding that patients may continue to inject drugs, harm reduction tools help providers propose realistic strategies to lower the chance of future complications, such as infections and overdose.

When treating PWID for an infection, screening for and addressing high-risk injection practices may help prevent future infections.[82] There are modifiable factors that can increase SSTI risk, including injection site, depth of injection, and setting in which people inject (eg, on the street, in a public bathroom, or in a supervised consumption site).[9,17,18,23,82,83] A 7-point risk score, the Bacterial Infectious Risk Scale for Injectors,[18] has been proposed as a potential tool for scoring risk of developing SSTI among PWID (**Box 1**). Skin-popping" or injection of drugs into subcutaneous tissue, can increase risk of bacterial infection (**Fig. 4**). Providers should first familiarize themselves with injection practices and be comfortable discussing injection habits with their patients (**Box 2, Table 1**). Several guides help outline safe injection practices with a harm reduction approach. The authors recommend the *Harm Reduction Coalition's Getting Off Right Safety* manual: https://harmreduction.org/wp-content/uploads/2011/12/getting-off-right.pdf. Increased uptake of safe injection equipment and medications for opioid use disorder has been demonstrated to decrease rates of SSTIs among people who use drugs.[84] A list of harm reduction practices for providers to be familiar with and able to discuss with patients is included in **Box 3**.

Identification and treatment of the infection are just the beginning of providing care. It is critical for PWID to have a timely linkage to substance use treatment, such as buprenorphine, methadone, or naltrexone, at the time of hospitalization, which has been shown to be feasible and beneficial.[85] Unfortunately, only a small subset of infectious diseases providers have been trained in the use of buprenorphine, and most patients do not have specific plans or recommendations for substance use disorder treatment upon discharge.[68] Inpatient addiction medicine or addiction psychiatry consultation is associated with better medical and substance use outcomes and fewer

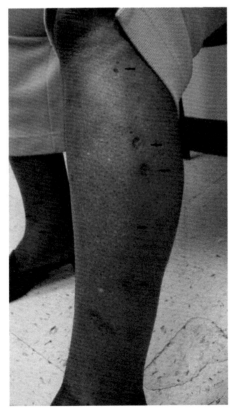

Fig. 4. Person with scars from skin-popping. (*From* Saporito R C, Lopez Pineiro M A, Migden M R, et al. (June 01, 2018) Recognizing Skin Popping Scars: A Complication of Illicit Drug Use. Cureus 2018;10(6): e2726).

Box 2
Providers should be comfortable asking about safe injection practices

Suggested Wording: "I want to make sure we treat your infection now and help prevent another infection from developing. Could you tell me a little about how you typically use?"

In the past month, how often have you shared needles or injection equipment with others?

In the past month, how often have you reused needles, cookers or filters? Where do you typically get water?

Do you rotate sites? Do you clean the site before injecting? Do you have alcohol pads?

Do you have access to clean injection supplies? Do you know where to find them?

---

readmissions.[86,87,88] Naloxone at time of discharge is a practice that may reduce fatalities from overdose.[89] Rapid fentanyl test strips (FTS) are used to detect fentanyl in illicit drugs and to help inform PWID about their risk of fentanyl exposure before consumption. FTS have shown a high level of acceptability and behavioral changes reported by users and may be a useful harm reduction intervention to reduce fentanyl overdose risk among this population.[90] In addition to treatment options for substance use disorder, providers should also be familiar with appropriate screening tests, vaccinations, and other medication options for PWID, including preexposure prophylaxis to prevent HIV (**Table 2**).

In addition to the barriers restricting access to clean injection supplies and medications, many structural elements also impede the ability of PWID to use safely. Among these, the criminalization and intense stigma associated with drug use render it physically difficult to use in a safe and dignified way. The consequence of "rushing" to inject has been described by PWID as a significant barrier to actually implementing these safe injection practices.[28] Fear of police encounters and housing insecurity, for example, can force individuals to rush while injecting and pose a challenge to implementing their knowledge of safe injection practices.[28] As a result, people are increasingly forced into public spaces to inject and placed at greater risk or injection-related harm in these environments.[83]

Table 1
Injection equipment: knowing the materials involved in can be helpful for discussing injection practices with patients

Equipment	Purpose
Cookers, that is, bottle caps, soda cans, spoons	Used to dissolve powdered and solid drugs
Filters, that is, cottons	Used to filter particulate matter when drawing up drug solution from cooker into syringe
Needle and syringe	To inject drugs
Water	To dissolve solid/powder drugs and to flush syringe
Tourniquets	To improve vein access
Acidifier, that is, vitamin C, vinegar	To help dissolve some drugs (ie, crack, black tar heroin)

Adapted from Principles of harm reduction. Harm Reduction Coalition. Newsline People AIDS Coalit N Y, 1998: p. 7-8 with permission.

Box 3
Harm reduction strategies for people who inject drugs

Injection materials
  Water: Encourage and provide access to sterile water as the safest choice. Other options
  include boiled water, then less preferably cold tap water (ie, sink or drinking fountain)
  Syringes: Ideal to use new syringe with each injection. If the patient reuses syringes,
  emphasize cleaning before reuse with one of the following:
  1. Cold water to rinse 3 times
  2. Undiluted bleach: shake for at least 2 minutes and discard; do this 3 times
  3. Cold water to rinse 3 times
  Provide access to clean syringes through referral to local syringe exchange program, safe
  injection kits, or by prescription to a pharmacy (ie, insulin syringes)
  Filters: Cotton balls, Q-tip cotton preferable to cigarette filters (which may contain
  particulate matter or contaminants)
  Acidifier: Used to dissolve some drugs, that is, crack cocaine or black tar heroin. Encourage
  (and if possible, provide) vitamin C powder as preferable to lemon juice or vinegar
  Alcohol swabs and hand sanitizer: provide before discharge

Injection practices
  Avoid sharing injection supplies with others and use new syringe for each injection
  If syringes must be reused, clean them thoroughly with cold water, then bleach, before use
  Use thinner (higher gauge) needles that create smaller holes and disrupt skin barrier less
  Avoid licking needle before injecting because this can introduce bacteria
  Wash hands or use hand sanitizer before injecting
  Use alcohol swabs to clean skin before injecting
  Avoid skin or muscle popping when injecting because this predisposes to abscess formation
  Rotate injection sites: Inject at least 1 inch from the last site to allow healing/prevent scarring
  Injection location: Avoid areas with higher bacterial burden and major arteries/nerves—
  order of preference: arms > back of hands > legs > feet > groin > neck
  Avoid injecting or using drugs alone
  Test dose: Try small amount of drug first to test its strength before using
  Have access to naloxone and be familiar with how to use
  Avoid sharpening needles as this can weaken the needle

Adapted from Principles of harm reduction. Harm Reduction Coalition. Newsline People AIDS
Coalit N Y, 1998: p. 7-8; with permission.

To combat these structural factors, new environments must be created for people to use drugs in a safe way.[91] The expansion of syringe exchange programs represents a critical intervention to broaden access to safe injection supplies and has been demonstrated to reduce the infectious complications associated with drug use.[92] Supervised consumption spaces are still not established in the United States and represent an unmet need in the response to substance use disorder treatment nationally. The

---

Table 2
Screening and treatment considerations for people who inject drugs

Screening	Vaccines	Medications
HIV	Influenza (yearly)	Medication for opioid use disorder
Hepatitis C	Hepatitis A and B	(buprenorphine, methadone,
Hepatitis B	Meningococcus (if housing	naltrexone ER)
GC/chlamydia	insecurity present)	HIV preexposure prophylaxis
Syphilis	Tdap (ensure updated every 10 y)	Naloxone
	PPSV-23	

Adapted from Massachusetts General Hospital Substance Use Disorder Curriculum: Harm Reduction for Providers; with permission.

establishment of these safe spaces would allow individuals to use under clinical supervision and have been demonstrated to reduce the harms associated with injection drug use, including SSTI.[93,94]

SUMMARY

PWID frequently engage in the health care system for the management of SSTIs and bone and joint infections. SSTIs have a wide variety of manifestations ranging from cellulitis to necrotizing fasciitis and can even resemble a vasculitis. The diagnosis of SSTIs is made by physical examination, and ultrasound can aid when the examination is equivocal for fluid collections. Up to 40% of SSTIs in PWID are polymicrobial. Gram positives and common commensal organisms of the oral cavity are frequently identified. Tissue/fluid cultures should be obtained to aid in antibiotic de-escalation. Blood cultures in SSTIs are of low yield. Surgical consultation should be obtained for deeper infections. Bone and joint infections are also frequently polymicrobial with a similar microbiologic pattern as SSTIs, and a higher prevalence of gram-negative and fungal pathogens. These infections typically require a prolonged course of antibiotics. Novel long-acting and oral antibiotic formulations have shown promising results particularly when barriers to compliance are identified. Further studies and innovative models are needed. PWID contacting the health care system should always be offered treatment for substance use disorder, counseling regarding high-risk injection practices, as well as appropriate screening, vaccines, and information surrounding harm reduction tools.

CLINICAL CARE POINTS

- Skin manifestations of injection drug use can be infectious and non-infectious, a thorough and non-judgmental history and physical exam is necessary.
- Whereas joint infections may present with overt signs, bone infections may present indolently and require a high index of suspicion.
- Clinicians should be comfortable discussing injection practices with patients in order to provide harm reduction counseling.
- Encounters with people who inject drugs for treatment of infections are also opportunities to engage in discussions about treatment for substance use disorder and pre-exposure prophylaxis for HIV.

DISCLOSURE

C.S. Saldana and D.A. Vyas have nothing to disclose. A.G. Wurcel received support from Merck.

REFERENCES

1. Ciccarone D, et al. Nationwide increase in hospitalizations for heroin-related soft tissue infections: associations with structural market conditions. Drug Alcohol Depend 2016;163:126–33.
2. Oh DHW, et al. Increased mortality and reoperation rates after treatment for septic arthritis of the knee in people who inject drugs: nationwide inpatient sample, 2000-2013. Clin Orthop Relat Res 2018;476(8):1557–65.
3. Kerr T, et al. High rates of primary care and emergency department use among injection drug users in Vancouver. J Public Health (Oxf) 2005;27(1):62–6.
4. Takahashi TA, et al. Predictors of hospitalization for injection drug users seeking care for soft tissue infections. J Gen Intern Med 2007;22(3):382–8.

5. Binswanger IA, et al. Drug users seeking emergency care for soft tissue infection at high risk for subsequent hospitalization and death. J Stud Alcohol Drugs 2008; 69(6):924–32.
6. Coughlin PA, Mavor AI. Arterial consequences of recreational drug use. Eur J Vasc Endovasc Surg 2006;32(4):389–96.
7. Raff AB, Kroshinsky D. Cellulitis: a review. JAMA 2016;316(3):325–37.
8. Abrahamian FM. Update: Clostridium novyi and unexplained illness among injecting-drug users–Scotland, Ireland, and England, April-June 2000. Ann Emerg Med 2001;37(1):107–9.
9. Murphy EL, et al. Risk factors for skin and soft-tissue abscesses among injection drug users: a case-control study. Clin Infect Dis 2001;33(1):35–40.
10. Heng MC, Feinberg M, Haberfelde G. Erythematous cutaneous nodules caused by adulterated cocaine. J Am Acad Dermatol 1989;21(3 Pt 1):570–2.
11. Redmond WJ. Heroin adulterants and skin disease. Arch Dermatol 1979; 115(1):111.
12. Bardenheier B, et al. Tetanus surveillance–United States, 1995-1997. MMWR CDC Surveill Summ 1998;47(2):1–13.
13. Passaro DJ, et al. Wound botulism associated with black tar heroin among injecting drug users. JAMA 1998;279(11):859–63.
14. Mars SG, et al. The textures of heroin: user perspectives on "black tar" and powder heroin in two U.S. cities. J Psychoactive Drugs 2016;48(4):270–8.
15. Frank RG, Pollack HA. Addressing the fentanyl threat to public health. N Engl J Med 2017;376(7):605–7.
16. Lambdin BH, et al. Associations between perceived illicit fentanyl use and infectious disease risks among people who inject drugs. Int J Drug Policy 2019;74: 299–304.
17. Hope V, et al. Frequency, factors and costs associated with injection site infections: findings from a national multi-site survey of injecting drug users in England. BMC Infect Dis 2008;8:120.
18. Phillips KT, Stein MD. Risk practices associated with bacterial infections among injection drug users in Denver, Colorado. Am J Drug Alcohol Abuse 2010; 36(2):92–7.
19. Kasper KJ, et al. A controlled-release oral opioid supports S. aureus survival in injection drug preparation equipment and may increase bacteremia and endocarditis risk. PLoS One 2019;14(8):e0219777.
20. Silverman M, et al. Hydromorphone and the risk of infective endocarditis among people who inject drugs: a population-based, retrospective cohort study. Lancet Infect Dis 2020;20(4):487–97.
21. Barocas JA, et al. Sociodemographic factors and social determinants associated with toxicology confirmed polysubstance opioid-related deaths. Drug Alcohol Depend 2019;200:59–63.
22. Hoots B, Vivolo-Kantor A, Seth P. The rise in non-fatal and fatal overdoses involving stimulants with and without opioids in the United States. Addiction 2020;115(5):946–58.
23. Dahlman D, et al. Both localized and systemic bacterial infections are predicted by injection drug use: a prospective follow-up study in Swedish criminal justice clients. PLoS One 2018;13(5):e0196944.
24. Abara WE, et al. Age-related differences in past or present hepatitis c virus infection among people who inject drugs: National Human Immunodeficiency Virus Behavioral Surveillance, 8 US Cities, 2015. J Infect Dis 2019;220(3):377–85.

25. Nerlander LMC, et al. HIV infection among MSM who inject methamphetamine in 8 US cities. Drug Alcohol Depend 2018;190:216–23.
26. Trayner KMA, et al. Increased risk of HIV and other drug-related harms associated with injecting in public places: national bio-behavioural survey of people who inject drugs. Int J Drug Policy 2020;77:102663.
27. Arendt V, et al. Injection of cocaine is associated with a recent HIV outbreak in people who inject drugs in Luxembourg. PLoS One 2019;14(5):e0215570.
28. Harris M, et al. Injecting-related health harms and overuse of acidifiers among people who inject heroin and crack cocaine in London: a mixed-methods study. Harm Reduct J 2019;16(1):60.
29. Bruckner JV, et al. Histopathological evaluation of cocaine-induced skin lesions in the rat. J Cutan Pathol 1982;9(2):83–95.
30. Mihu MR, et al. Methamphetamine alters the antimicrobial efficacy of phagocytic cells during methicillin-resistant Staphylococcus aureus skin infection. mBio 2015;6(6). e01622-15.
31. Darke S, Ross J, Kaye S. Physical injecting sites among injecting drug users in Sydney, Australia. Drug Alcohol Depend 2001;62(1):77–82.
32. Martin H, et al. Characteristics of chronic wounds in substance abuse: a retrospective study of 58 patients. Ann Dermatol Venereol 2019;146(12):793–800 [in French].
33. Smith DJ Jr, et al. Drug injection injuries of the upper extremity. Ann Plast Surg 1989;22(1):19–24.
34. Pieper B, Templin T. Chronic venous insufficiency in persons with a history of injection drug use. Res Nurs Health 2001;24(5):423–32.
35. Lindell TD, Porter JM, Langston C. Intra-arterial injections of oral medications. A complication of drug addiction. N Engl J Med 1972;287(22):1132–3.
36. Wilson RM, Elmaraghi S, Rinker BD. Ischemic hand complications from intra-arterial injection of sublingual buprenorphine/naloxone among patients with opioid dependency. Hand (N Y) 2017;12(5):507–11.
37. al Zahrani HA. Vascular complications following intravascular self-injection of addictive drugs. J R Coll Surg Edinb 1997;42(1):50–3.
38. Abidin MR, et al. Injection of illicit drugs into the granulation tissue of chronic ulcers. Ann Plast Surg 1990;24(3):268–70.
39. Ciccarone D, Harris M. Fire in the vein: heroin acidity and its proximal effect on users' health. Int J Drug Policy 2015;26(11):1103–10.
40. Kazlouskaya V, et al. A case of heroin linear track hyperpigmentation: histopathology and treatment with Q-switched Nd:YAG 1064nm laser. Int J Dermatol 2018; 57(3):362–4.
41. Hennings C, Miller J. Illicit drugs: what dermatologists need to know. J Am Acad Dermatol 2013;69(1):135–42.
42. Korantzopoulos P, et al. Atrial fibrillation and marijuana smoking. Int J Clin Pract 2008;62(2):308–13.
43. Grund JP, Latypov A, Harris M. Breaking worse: the emergence of krokodil and excessive injuries among people who inject drugs in Eurasia. Int J Drug Policy 2013;24(4):265–74.
44. Auffenberg C, Rosenthal LJ, Dresner N. Levamisole: a common cocaine adulterant with life-threatening side effects. Psychosomatics 2013;54(6):590–3.
45. Tran H, Tan D, Marnejon TP. Cutaneous vasculopathy associated with levamisole-adulterated cocaine. Clin Med Res 2013;11(1):26–30.
46. Peterson TC, et al. Septic arthritis in intravenous drug abusers: a historical comparison of habits and pathogens. J Emerg Med 2014;47(6):723–8.

47. Reinus WR, De Cotiis D, Schaffer A. Changing patterns of septic tenosynovitis of the distal extremities. Emerg Radiol 2015;22(2):133–9.
48. Gomez-Rodriguez N, et al. [Infectious bursitis: study of 40 cases in the pre-patellar and olecranon regions]. Enferm Infecc Microbiol Clin 1997;15(5):237–42.
49. Chandrasekar PH, Narula AP. Bone and joint infections in intravenous drug abusers. Rev Infect Dis 1986;8(6):904–11.
50. Sapico FL, Montgomerie JZ. Vertebral osteomyelitis in intravenous drug abusers: report of three cases and review of the literature. Rev Infect Dis 1980;2(2):196–206.
51. Roca RP, Yoshikawa TT. Primary skeletal infections in heroin users: a clinical characterization, diagnosis and therapy. Clin Orthop Relat Res 1979;(144):238–48.
52. Gordon RJ, Lowy FD. Bacterial infections in drug users. N Engl J Med 2005;353(18):1945–54.
53. Voon P, et al. Denial of prescription analgesia among people who inject drugs in a Canadian setting. Drug Alcohol Rev 2015;34(2):221–8.
54. Khan IA, Vaccaro AR, Zlotolow DA. Management of vertebral diskitis and osteomyelitis. Orthopedics 1999;22(8):758–65.
55. Jenkins TC, et al. Microbiology and initial antibiotic therapy for injection drug users and non-injection drug users with cutaneous abscesses in the era of community-associated methicillin-resistant Staphylococcus aureus. Acad Emerg Med 2015;22(8):993–7.
56. Allison DC, et al. Microbiology of bone and joint infections in injecting drug abusers. Clin Orthop Relat Res 2010;468(8):2107–12.
57. Summanen PH, et al. Bacteriology of skin and soft-tissue infections: comparison of infections in intravenous drug users and individuals with no history of intravenous drug use. Clin Infect Dis 1995;20(Suppl 2):S279–82.
58. Stenstrom R, et al. Prevalence of and risk factors for methicillin-resistant Staphylococcus aureus skin and soft tissue infection in a Canadian emergency department. CJEM 2009;11(5):430–8.
59. Young DM, et al. An epidemic of methicillin-resistant Staphylococcus aureus soft tissue infections among medically underserved patients. Arch Surg 2004;139(9):947–51 [discussion: 951–3].
60. Talan DA, Summanen PH, Finegold SM. Ampicillin/sulbactam and cefoxitin in the treatment of cutaneous and other soft-tissue abscesses in patients with or without histories of injection drug abuse. Clin Infect Dis 2000;31(2):464–71.
61. Ghasemi Barghi R, Mirakbari SM. Septic arthritis of sternoclavicular joint: a case report of a rare finding in injecting drug users. Arch Iran Med 2010;13(3):248–50.
62. Stevens DL, et al. Practice guidelines for the diagnosis and management of skin and soft tissue infections: 2014 update by the Infectious Diseases Society of America. Clin Infect Dis 2014;59(2):e10–52.
63. Subramaniam S, et al. Point-of-care ultrasound for diagnosis of abscess in skin and soft tissue infections. Acad Emerg Med 2016;23(11):1298–306.
64. Torres J, et al. Low yield of blood and wound cultures in patients with skin and soft-tissue infections. Am J Emerg Med 2017;35(8):1159–61.
65. Perl B, et al. Cost-effectiveness of blood cultures for adult patients with cellulitis. Clin Infect Dis 1999;29(6):1483–8.
66. Hassan AS, et al. Peripheral bacterial septic arthritis: review of diagnosis and management. J Clin Rheumatol 2017;23(8):435–42.
67. Brook I. Microbiology and management of joint and bone infections due to anaerobic bacteria. J Orthopaedic Sci 2008;13(2):169.

68. Rapoport AB, et al. Infectious diseases physicians' perspectives regarding injection drug use and related infections, United States, 2017. Open Forum Infect Dis 2018;5(7):ofy132.
69. Suzuki J, et al. Outpatient parenteral antimicrobial therapy among people who inject drugs: a review of the literature. Open Forum Infect Dis 2018;5(9):ofy194.
70. Serota DP, Vettese T. New answers for old questions in the treatment of severe infections from injection drug use. J Hosp Med 2019;14:e1–7.
71. Eaton EF, et al. A 9-point risk assessment for patients who inject drugs and require intravenous antibiotics: focusing inpatient resources on patients at greatest risk of ongoing drug use. Clin Infect Dis 2019;68(6):1041–3.
72. Fanucchi LC, et al. Outpatient parenteral antimicrobial therapy plus buprenorphine for opioid use disorder and severe injection-related infections. Clin Infect Dis 2020;70(6):1226–9.
73. Li HK, et al. Oral versus intravenous antibiotics for bone and joint infection. N Engl J Med 2019;380(5):425–36.
74. Overcash JS, O'Riordan W, Quintas M, et al. 470. Treatment of acute bacterial skin and skin structure infections (ABSSSI) in patients with significant drug abuse: outcomes from global phase 3 studies of delafloxacin (DLX). Open Forum Infect Dis 2019;6:S230.
75. Gonzalez PL, et al. Treatment of acute bacterial skin and skin structure infection with single-dose dalbavancin in persons who inject drugs. Drugs Context 2018;7: 212559.
76. Bryson-Cahn C, et al. Dalbavancin as secondary therapy for serious Staphylococcus aureus infections in a vulnerable patient population. Open Forum Infect Dis 2019;6(2):ofz028.
77. Tirupathi R, et al. Acute bacterial skin and soft tissue infections: new drugs in ID armamentarium. J Community Hosp Intern Med Perspect 2019;9(4):310–3.
78. Gilbert AR, et al. Self-care habits among people who inject drugs with skin and soft tissue infections: a qualitative analysis. Harm Reduct J 2019;16(1):69.
79. Harris RE, et al. Experiences with skin and soft tissue infections among people who inject drugs in Philadelphia: a qualitative study. Drug Alcohol Depend 2018;187:8–12.
80. Monteiro J, et al. Self-treatment of skin infections by people who inject drugs. Drug Alcohol Depend 2020;206:107695.
81. Principles of harm reduction. Harm reduction coalition. Newsline People AIDS Coalit N Y, 1998: p. 7–8.
82. Phillips KT, et al. Skin and needle hygiene intervention for injection drug users: results from a randomized, controlled stage I pilot trial. J Subst Abuse Treat 2012;43(3):313–21.
83. Small W, et al. Public injection settings in Vancouver: physical environment, social context and risk. Int J Drug Policy 2007;18(1):27–36.
84. Dunleavy K, et al. Association between harm reduction intervention uptake and skin and soft tissue infections among people who inject drugs. Drug Alcohol Depend 2017;174:91–7.
85. Liebschutz JM, et al. Buprenorphine treatment for hospitalized, opioid-dependent patients: a randomized clinical trial. JAMA Intern Med 2014;174(8):1369–76.
86. Degenhardt L, et al. Global patterns of opioid use and dependence: harms to populations, interventions, and future action. Lancet 2019;394(10208):1560–79.
87. Wakeman SE, Metlay JP, Chang Y, et al. Inpatient addiction consultation for hospitalized patients increases post-discharge. abstinence and reduces addiction severity. J Gen Intern Med 2017;32(8):909–16.

88. Trowbridge P, Weinstein ZM, Kerensky T, et al. Addiction consultation services - Linking hospitalized patients to outpatient addiction treatment. J Subst Abuse Treat 2017;79:1–5.
89. Mueller SR, et al. A review of opioid overdose prevention and naloxone prescribing: implications for translating community programming into clinical practice. Subst Abus 2015;36(2):240–53.
90. Goldman JE, et al. Perspectives on rapid fentanyl test strips as a harm reduction practice among young adults who use drugs: a qualitative study. Harm Reduct J 2019;16(1):3.
91. McGowan CR, et al. Risk environments and the ethics of reducing drug-related harms. Am J Bioeth 2017;17(12):46–8.
92. Bhattacharya MK, et al. Impact of a harm-reduction programme on soft tissue infections among injecting drug users of Kolkata, India. J Health Popul Nutr 2006; 24(1):121–2.
93. Irwin A, et al. A cost-benefit analysis of a potential supervised injection facility in San Francisco, California, USA. J Drug Issues 2017;47(2):164–84.
94. Potier C, et al. Supervised injection services: what has been demonstrated? A systematic literature review. Drug Alcohol Depend 2014;145:48–68.

Management of Opioid Use Disorder and Infectious Disease in the Inpatient Setting

Ellen F. Eaton, MD, MSPH[a],*, Theresa Vettese, MD[b],*

KEYWORDS

• Injection drug use • Opioids • Medications for opioid use disorder

KEY POINTS

- Hospitals and acute care physicians have an important role in diagnosing and treating opioid use disorder (OUD).
- Medications for OUD is the cornerstone of care for persons with OUD and should be promptly initiated in acute and primary health care settings.
- Reducing pain, withdrawal, and stigma for persons with OUD is essential for a therapeutic hospital experience and promotes engagement in care.

INTRODUCTION

Although opioid use disorder (OUD) is a chronic disease, it is associated with many acute and life-threatening complications that are increasingly common driving high rates of opioid-related hospitalization.[1,2] Since the opioid crisis began, the number of persons seeking emergency care and/or hospitalized annually for overdose, trauma, and severe infections is rising.[3,4] Of those with OUD, persons who inject opioids are most vulnerable to these conditions because of injection-related behaviors and the frequency of injection in opioid dependency, which increases the risk of infection and overdose.[5,6] This article focuses on inpatient care as an important opportunity to reach, engage, and treat persons with OUD. Unlike acute care, outpatient care and preventive services for harm reduction and infection prevention are not frequently used by substance-using patients.[7] Poverty, rurality, lack of insurance, and stigma are among the reasons that persons with OUD do not seek medical care until they are very ill.[7] Many patients are uninsured, rural, or stigmatized, and their drug use behaviors are often criminalized.[8,9] These factors preclude them from engaging in

[a] Division of Infectious Disease, University of Alabama at Birmingham, 845 19th Street South, Birmingham, AL 35205, USA; [b] Division of General Medicine and Geriatrics, Emory University School of Medicine, 49 Jesse Hill Drive, Atlanta, GA 30303, USA
* Corresponding authors.
E-mail addresses: eeaton@uab.edu (E.F.E.); tvettes@emory.edu (T.V.)
Twitter: @DrEllenEaton (E.F.E.); @TracyVettese (T.V.)

Infect Dis Clin N Am 34 (2020) 511–524
https://doi.org/10.1016/j.idc.2020.06.008
0891-5520/20/© 2020 Elsevier Inc. All rights reserved.
id.theclinics.com

community-based care to prevent serious complications of OUD including infection and overdose. Hospitalizations is, therefore, increasingly a touch-point for patients with OUD.[10]

HISTORY

The United States is nearly 3 decades into the opioid epidemic. In recent history, the public health burden of OUD has become so great that annual opioid overdose fatalities exceed the AIDS epidemic, even at its peak, by tens of thousands of deaths per year.[11] As of 2016, 2.1 million people in the United States had OUD according to the National Institute on Drug Abuse.[12] Yet, only 20% of these individuals receive treatment based on national estimates.[12] The number of opioid-related deaths is unacceptable: opioids accounted for 68,000 deaths in 2018 and more than 700,000 since 1999.[13] This highlights the urgent need to link and engage persons with OUD to evidence-based treatment, including medications for OUD (MOUD), as soon as possible for harm reduction and to promote engagement in treatment of other medical conditions, such as infectious diseases.

Reports from Centers for Disease Control and Prevention and Substance Abuse and Mental Health Services Administration indicate that rural and Southern states are disproportionately affected by the opioid epidemic.[13] Relative to urban areas, many rural regions also have higher opioid prescribing rates. In 2017, residents of Alabama, Tennessee, Kentucky, Mississippi, Louisiana, Arkansas, and Oklahoma received 83 or more opioid prescriptions per 100 residents; the national average was 58.7.[14] Not surprisingly, Appalachian states continue to have the highest rate of opioid-related Emergency Department and hospital admission rates.[15] From 1999 to 2015, opioid-related deaths in young rural people (18–25 years) quadrupled; deaths among women tripled.[16] Lack of access to evidence-based treatment, such as addiction treatment providers and MOUD, and restrictions on harm reduction policies, including syringe service programs, have led to poor outcomes in rural areas. Thus, persons who use illicit drugs remain untreated and hard to reach due to stigma, poverty, and rurality.

DEFINITIONS

OUD is defined as a problematic pattern of opioid use resulting in clinically significant impairment per the DSM-5 criteria. In general, OUD consists of the 3 "Cs": loss of Control, adverse Consequences (health, legal, relationships), and Cravings for the substance. An affirmative response to 2 or more criteria is consistent with a diagnosis of OUD.

MOUD include methadone, buprenorphine, and naltrexone, which are approved by Food and Drug Administration for the treatment of OUD.[12]

BACKGROUND

The clinical and economic burden that the opioid crisis has placed on hospitals cannot be understated. Admissions for persons who inject drugs are among the costliest and lengthy.[17,18] Because persons who inject drugs (PWID) often have multiple comorbidities (eg, mental health disorders) and lack insurance and social support, they receive inpatient care for conditions that may otherwise be cared for in the home with support services such as home health nursing or physical therapy.[19] Blood stream infections, endocarditis, bone, joint, skin, and soft tissue infections are all common infections among hospitalized PWID that may require parenteral antibiotics in conjunction with surgery, wound care, and physical rehabilitation. Yet, once acute issues have stabilized, most clinicians do not transition PWID to an unsupervised outpatient setting (eg, home) for outpatient parenteral antibiotics for PWID.[20] Although there is emerging data that outpatient parenteral antibiotic therapy (OPAT) is safe and effective in PWID, many clinicians cite concerns about medication adherence and substance use as barriers to OPAT for PWID. Thus, hospitalized persons with these infections may remain hospitalized for the duration of their care, which may be weeks to months of pharmacotherapy, surgical interventions, and wound care.[21] The average length of stay for hospitalized PWID with infections ranges from 15 to 38 days.[19,21] Not surprisingly, PWID with endocarditis have a longer length of stay and more readmissions relative to patients without a history of intravenous drug use.[22]

SCREENING FOR OPIOD USE DISORDER IN THE HOSPITAL SETTING

Following an increase of OUD nationally along with OUD-related complications, the US Preventive Services Task Force and National Institute on Drug Abuse recommend that all adults receive screening for illicit drug use. This is especially important in acute care settings, which may be the only health care setting in which patients with OUD seek care due to the life-threatening nature of overdose, accidents, or infection. For this reason, the authors recommend that clinicians in all inpatient settings operationalize screening for illicit drug use such that it becomes part of routine clinical care.

There are multiple validated screening tools, but given time constraints in the acute care setting, the authors advocate use of the Rapid Opioid Dependence Screen (RODS), an 8-item measure of opioid dependence that can be conducted in less than 5 minutes and has been demonstrated to be highly accurate.[23] If patients screen positive for opioid dependence using the RODS tool, clinicians should proceed to confirm OUD using the 2013 *Diagnostic and Statistical Manual of Mental Disorders* of the American Psychiatric Association criteria for OUD.[24] In patients who meet the criteria for OUD, additional substance use history should be obtained, including what substances are used, frequency of consumption, amount consumed, problematic consequences of use, treatment history, and age at first use.

The amount and type of opioids used influences the likelihood and severity of withdrawal symptoms and the approach to acute pain management. Thus, it is useful to obtain additional information regarding quantity, frequency, and number of times per day opioids are used. In the Eastern United States heroin users often describe their quantity of use in number of "bags." One "bag" of heroin is approximately 100 mg of retail heroin. In the Western United States users will usually describe quantity in fractions of a gram. On average, heroin sold retail in the United States is 33% pure; the remainder added adulterants.[25] Cost can also be used to estimate quantity of heroin use. The 2018 Drug Enforcement Administration data reveal an average cost of 900 dollars per pure gram or between 5 and 20 dollars per "bag" retail. It is challenging to convert illicit heroin to morphine equivalents, as one must consider the wide variation in purity and understand that the stated use of heroin (eg, 500 mg daily) reflects weight and not dosage. Considering previous data and average purity, the parenteral morphine equivalent to a "bag" of heroin (100 mg) is approximately 15 to 30 mg.

Obtaining additional history regarding other substance use is also important since alcohol and benzodiazepine withdrawal can be life threatening, and methamphetamine use (including injection) has become increasingly prevalent across the United States.

ROLE OF ADDICTION MEDICINE CONSULTATION

Once identified, persons with OUD should be referred to a provider with expertise in Addiction Medicine. In the inpatient setting, addiction medicine providers serve an invaluable role. Marks and colleagues[26] demonstrated that addiction medicine consultation was significantly associated with MOUD receipt. Addiction medicine consultation may improve other hospital outcomes as well: reducing readmissions, discharges against medical advice (AMA), and elopements, and increasing the odds of antibiotic completion for persons with infections.[26] But, addiction medicine expertise is not necessary to initiate medications for OUD. In fact, recent reports by the Institute for Healthcare Improvement and the National Academy of Medicine call for Infectious Diseases and other providers without training in addiction medicine to take an active role in the treatment of OUD.[27,28] However, busy clinicians need support in order to obtain the requisite training for buprenorphine prescribing. Health systems can support these clinicians and expand their OUD treatment workforce by sponsoring the requisite training to prescribe buprenorphine (ie, Drug Addiction Treatment Act [DATA]-waived).[29] This may mean the health systems bring on-site training to the hospitals and give clinicians paid time off to obtain the 8-hour training requirements.

TREATMENT OF OPIOD USE DISORDER AND OPIOID WITHDRAWAL SYMPTOMS IN THE HOSPITAL

Any management of an IDU-associated infection is incomplete without addressing the underlying substance use disorder. Addiction is highly undertreated among patients with IDU-associated infections, which may contribute to poor infection-related outcomes.[30,31] Opioid agonist therapy with buprenorphine or methadone to prevent withdrawal should be routinely offered to all hospitalized patients with OUD including those with infectious complications of OUD with the goal of facilitating medical treatment and engaging patients in long-term treatment of their substance use disorder. Because extended release naltrexone administration requires complete detoxification from opioids, it is not appropriate for use in the hospital setting for patients with active OUD. Withdrawal symptoms in patients using short-acting opioids such as heroin begin in 6 to 12 hours after the last dose, peak in 36 to 72 hours, and last for 7 to 10 days. The severity of opioid withdrawal can be classified using the validated Clinical Opioid Withdrawal Scale.[32] When choosing between methadone and buprenorphine, one should consider patient preference, availability of outpatient treatment providers, comorbid medical conditions, and adverse effects.

Referral to addiction treatment has been associated with improved IDU-related infectious endocarditis (IE) mortality.[33] Initiation of MOUD can be achieved successfully in the emergency department, inpatient wards, and specifically in patients admitted with IDU-IE.[34–36] Protocols and resources for inpatient management of withdrawal and initiation of MOUD are available along with telephone support services for providers seeking guidance on specific cases.[33,37,38] Inpatient addiction consult services are an important resource for the management of hospitalized patients with OUD[39] and are associated with increased completion of antibiotics, decreased AMA discharge, and increased rates of MOUD provision among patients with IDU-associated infections.[40] However, when unavailable, initiation of opioid agonist therapy does not require an addiction specialist. Although buprenorphine prescribing in the outpatient setting requires certification, inpatient physicians are exempt from these requirements and can prescribe buprenorphine or methadone in the hospital setting.[41] In the outpatient setting, buprenorphine prescription is restricted to providers with a DATA of 2000 waiver, also known as an "X-waiver." X-waiver trainings last for 8 hours, and free web-based trainings are available.[42] At the time of discharge, non–X-waivered physicians can prescribe up to 72 hours of buprenorphine as a bridge to follow-up with outpatient addiction services.[43,44] In the outpatient setting, methadone can only be obtained through federally regulated methadone maintenance programs. Although linkage to care as an outpatient is ideal, opioid agonist therapy initiated in the hospital can be tapered before discharge if it is unavailable. Because of the duration of the acute phase of opioid withdrawal, a 7- to 10-day taper is preferred, but tapering can be safely done over 3 to 5 days if needed.[38] **Fig. 1** outlines the initiation of methadone or buprenorphine for the treatment of both withdrawal and OUD in the inpatient setting.

Although not as effective as opioid agonist therapy, alpha-adrenergic agonists and other nonopioid agents can be useful adjuncts in treating symptoms of opioid withdrawal (**Table 1**).

HARM REDUCTION

Harm reduction involves "meeting people where they are" and providing services they are willing to accept with the goal of improving their health or preventing negative outcomes including unintentional overdose and infectious complications. One important aspect of reducing harm involves maintaining patients in care for their concomitant OUD and infection, ideally avoiding AMA discharge. In one cohort of patients admitted with IDU-associated infections, 49% of those without an addiction medicine consult left by patient-directed discharge (PDD), also known as against medical advice.[40] In hospitalizations in which patients with OUD are administered methadone for prevention of withdrawal, there is a significant reduction in AMA discharges.[45] Opioid agonist treatment may also lead to decreased surreptitious drug use in the hospital.[41] If a patient plans to leave AMA, all efforts should be made to provide them with oral antibiotics that might be effective, even if suboptimal, for their infection. Inpatient physicians should consider documenting an oral "antibiotic contingency plan" that can be rapidly enacted if a patient is imminently leaving the hospital. The patient leaving AMA should be provided with outpatient follow-up appointments with infectious disease or primary care. All patients with IDU-associated infections should be discharged with naloxone, overdose prevention education, and community resources for addiction treatment and syringe exchange programs.

Physicians should appreciate the multiple steps in preparing opioids such as heroin and fentanyl for injection and the potential infectious risk: dissolving powder in a cooker, drawing the drug into a needle with syringe with/without a filter to strain out large matter, removing air bubbles from the syringe, and injection with or without aspiration of blood (confirmation of needle location). Acid may be used to assist with dissolving the drug. Acidification with citrus juices has been associated with candidiasis infection.[46] Patients who lick the needle before injection may develop streptococcus and anaerobic infections from their own oral flora.[47] If patients are injecting in femoral or lower extremity veins, they are at risk for gram-negative and anaerobic infections.[47] If they inject into subcutaneous tissues or muscles "skin popping," they are at risk for abscesses including spore-forming bacterial such as *Clostridum* and *Bacillus* species. Patients may aspirate blood into the needle tip via the syringe to confirm entry into the vessel before injecting the drug to confirm placement. This process will bring any blood-borne infections such as human immunodeficiency virus (HIV), hepatitis C virus, and hepatitis B virus into the syringe, and potentially transmit the infection if the syringe or other infected materials are reused. By inquiring about how patients use drugs, physicians can then educate patients on ways to reduce harm.

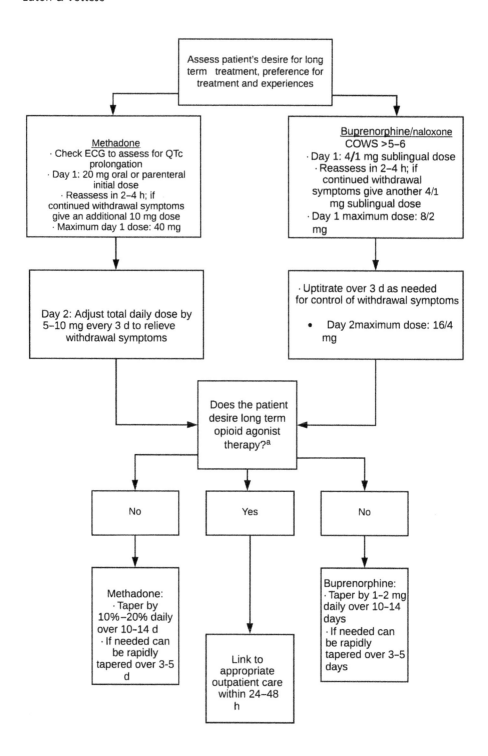

During admission, providers can give essential education on safe injection practices. Patients should be counseled to use an alcohol swab to sterilize the skin before infection.[48] This can reduce the likelihood of infection. Reusing drug-related materials is never recommended. However, patients who inject drugs can be counseled to use undiluted household bleach to sterilize drug use materials when reuse is expected. The drug use materials should be retained in bleach for at least 2 minutes.[49] Because HIV is effectively transmitted through shared syringes and other "works," HIV preexposure prophylaxis (PrEP) is recommended for persons who inject drugs. Patients who inject drugs may meet criteria for PrEP if they have specific drug sue behaviors including injecting with a partner with HIV infection, sharing injection equipment, and injecting despite recently receiving drug treatment. Many PWID who meet this criterion receive care in the hospital setting due to the infectious complications of injection. Therefore, the hospital is an ideal place to educate patients on HIV prevention and prescribe PrEP. Although PrEP uptake among PWID has been poor, leveraging a hospital harm reduction philosophy can allow eligible patients to receive important education and PrEP prescription. Physicians in acute care settings should consider other aspects of preventive care for persons with OUD who may not have access to routine medical care. Vaccination for influenza, pneumococcus, hepatitis A, and B can be achieved during the admission.

PAIN MANAGEMENT IN PATIENTS WITH OPIOID USE DISORDER
Patients with Active Opioid Use Disorder

In the hospital setting, patients with a history of active OUD often have their acute pain undertreated. This may be due to providers' misconceptions regarding pain and behavior in persons with OUD, including worrying that the patient's pain is exaggerated in order to obtain drugs, thinking that a regular opioid habit eliminates pain, believing that opioid therapy is not effective in patients with OUD, or worrying that prescribing opioids will exacerbate drug addiction. Data demonstrate that the presence of opioid addiction seems to worsen the experience of acute pain. These patients also often have a higher tolerance and thus require higher dosages and more frequent dosing of opioids to adequately treat their pain.[50]

In patients with OUD who have moderate-to-severe acute pain in the hospital, the management goal should be to improve function, quality of life, and prevent withdrawal symptoms and retain the patient in care. In communicating with a patient with OUD with severe acute pain, it is best to outline the pain management plan at admission, including the plan to manage the patient's acute pain, prevent opioid withdrawal symptoms, change to oral opioid analgesics as soon as possible, discussion of nonopioid and nondrug treatments, reinforcement that opioids will be tapered as the acute pain episode resolves, and a detailed plan for discharge.

One treatment strategy is to initiate methadone in split dosages (analgesic effect is lost with 24-hour dosing) with additional short-acting opioids titrated to pain. For

◄─────────────────────────────────────

Fig. 1. Treatment of patients with OUD undergoing withdrawal. [a] Long-term opioid agonist therapy is preferred and should be strongly encouraged. Buprenorphine can result in opioid withdrawal and should be used only in patients with clear evidence of mild to moderate opioid withdrawal. Methadone should be used with caution in patients with QTc prolongation. (*Data from* Rosenthal ES, Karchmer AW, Theisen-Toupal J, et al. Suboptimal addiction interventions for patients hospitalized with injection drug use-associated infective endocarditis. Am J Med. 2016;129(5):481-485; and Wesson DR, Ling W. The clinical opiate withdrawal scale (COWS). J Psychoactive Drugs. 2003;35(2):253-259.)

Table 1
Signs and symptoms of opioid withdrawal and nonopioid adjuvant treatments

Sign or Symptom	Pharmacologic Management
Tachycardia, hypertension, hyperthermia, diaphoresis, lacrimation, rhinorrhea, piloerection, mydriasis, yawning	Clonidine, 0.1-0.2 mg, orally every 4–6 h, daily maximum dose of 1.2 mg on day 1 and 2.0 mg afterward
Anxiety, insomnia	Antihistamine (eg, diphenhydramine), sedating antidepressant (eg, trazadone)
Myalgia, bone pain	Acetaminophen, nonsteroidal antiinflammatory (eg, ibuprofen)
Nausea and vomiting	Antiemetic (eg, prochlorperazine, ondansetron)
Diarrhea	Antidiarrheal (eg, loperamide)

patients unable to take oral agents, intravenous methadone is available and dosed at equivalent dosages. An alternative strategy is to initiate sublingual buprenorphine in split dosages.[51] These approaches are outlined in **Box 1**. Either strategy is effective at treating both the patient's pain and OUD, and, as in the case of treatment of OUD and withdrawal, one should consider patient preference, availability of outpatient treatment providers, comorbid medical conditions, and adverse effects. Alternatively, regularly scheduled short-acting opioids can be used alone but may lead to more withdrawal symptoms between dosages.[38]

Patients Receiving Opioid Agonist Therapy

When treating severe acute pain in patients receiving opioid agonist therapy for OUD, the methadone or buprenorphine dose should first be verified with the prescribing

Box 1
Opioid pain management for patients with active opiod use disorder and severe acute pain

Methadone:
- Check electrocardiogram to evaluate for QTC prolongation
- Day 1: methadone, 10 mg, orally q 8 hours with short-acting opioid analgesic PRN
- Methadone can be given intravenously if patient not able to take oral
- Patients may require increased and more frequent doses of short-acting opioid analgesics to achieve adequate pain control
- Taper short-acting opioid as patient clinically improves
- Discharge goal is daily dosing of methadone and immediate follow-up at methadone opioid treatment program or methadone taper over 7 to 10 days

Buprenorphine/naloxone:
- COWS >5 to 6
- Day 1: 2/.5 mg sublingual q 6 hours
- Day 2: 4/1 mg sublingual q 6 hours if patient still having severe pain or cravings/withdrawal symptoms and not sedated
- Can increase by 4/1 mg sublingual daily to maximum dose of 32/8 mg SL daily
- Discharge goal is daily dosing of buprenorphine/naloxone and immediate follow-up with buprenorphine provider or taper over 7 to 10 days

Abbreviations: COWS, Clinical Opiate Withdrawal Scale; PRN, as needed.

methadone clinic or physician. In addition, involving the patient in the decision process regarding pain management is essential. As in all cases of acute pain, nonopioid treatments should be a component of the pain management plan. It is important to understand that patients receiving opioid agonists for OUD are usually treated with one dose every 24 to 48 hours and do not receive sustained analgesia. In the case of patients on methadone as an MOUD, methadone should be continued at the prescribed daily dose and additional short-acting opioid analgesics should be given to provide appropriate pain relief. The methadone dose can be administered in split dosages to enhance analgesic effect. Because of opioid tolerance, patients receiving MOUD often require increased and more frequent doses of short-acting opioid analgesics to achieve adequate pain control.

Buprenorphine is a mu-opioid receptor partial agonist with high affinity for the mu-opioid receptor. Despite this, additional receptors remain available for full opioid agonists to bind to, and there is no need to discontinue buprenorphine when using additional opioid analgesics. An appropriate pain management strategy in these patients is to continue maintenance therapy with buprenorphine and treat acute pain with additional short-acting opioid agonists. Higher doses of opioid agonists and more frequent dosing may be needed to provide adequate pain relief, and opioids with higher affinity for the mu receptor (morphine, hydromorphone, fentanyl) may be more efficacious. As in the case with methadone, a split dose buprenorphine regimen will provide greater analgesia and may lower the requirements for additional opioids. **Box 2** provides examples of opioid dosing strategies in patients on MOUD.

Creating a Patient-Centered Environment for Persons with Opiod Use Disorder

It is important for clinicians and administrators to appreciate that for many persons with OUD, the hospital serves as a "risk environment."[52] Because of factors outside

---

Box 2
Opioid pain management for patients with severe acute pain on opioid agonist therapy

Patient taking buprenorphine/naloxone, 16/4 mg, SL daily for MOUD with acute severe pain:

- Verify dose with provider
- Buprenorphine/naloxone, 4/1 mg, SL q 6 hours and short-acting opioid agonist PRN
- Patients may require increased and more frequent doses of short-acting opioid analgesics to achieve adequate pain control
- Discharge goal is to taper off short-acting opioid and resume once daily buprenorphine dosing

Patient taking methadone, 90 mg, daily for MOUD with acute severe pain:

- Verify dose with methadone opioid treatment program
- Methadone, 30 mg, po (or intravenous if unable to take oral) q 8 hours and short-acting opioid agonist PRN
- Patients may require increased and more frequent doses of short-acting opioid analgesics to achieve adequate pain control
- Discharge goal is to taper off short-acting opioid agonist and resume once daily methadone dosing

Abbreviation: PRN, as needed.

of a patient's control, such as stigma and judgment from nursing staff and clinicians, patient may receive delayed or inappropriate treatment of pain, opioid withdrawal, and other symptoms. This suboptimal care makes it hard for patients to engage in their treatment plan for hospitalization.[45] If patients feel stigma from health care providers, it is unlikely that they will participate actively in their care including OUD treatment or discuss drug cravings and risk behaviors that merit further evaluation and education (eg, sharing needles).[53] Negative interactions with staff, untreated withdrawal and pain, and restrictive hospital policies have been associated with patient-directed discharge (PDD) or prematurely leaving the hospital, which is also known as "AMA."[54] This is an important outcome, as PDD is associated with increased mortality.[55,56] In one Canadian study evaluating all patients who leave via PDD, there was a 3-fold higher risk of death for patients with PDD in the year following admission relative to patients who did not leave early.[55] There was also a statistically larger percentage of persons who inject drugs among those leaving by PDD (54%) relative to those who did not (23%, $P<.001$). In addition to PDD, hospitalized PWID are at greater risk of inpatient illicit drug use, overdose, and death.[21,57] In-hospital illicit drug use is also common among persons who use drugs and leads to worsened stigma, shame, and even criminalization.[21] Yet, patients report using drugs to manage pain and withdrawal because these symptoms, when untreated, interfered with their medical treatment.[52] Thus talking openly about substance use behaviors and cravings, together with effective treatment of OUD, can promote healing and prevent high-risk illicit drug use behaviors. Finally, training all hospital staff to reduce stigma and support patient-centered care is essential to retain persons with OUD in care and reduce PDD.[9,52]

CLINICS CARE POINTS

- The hospital and emergency department setting provides a unique opportunity to diagnose and treat OUD
- All patients receiving acute care services should be screened for OUD
- Rapid opioid dependence screen, an 8- item measure of opioid dependence, which can be conducted in less than 5 minutes and has been demonstrated to be highly accurate
- All hospitalized patients with OUD who are not engaged in care should receive an addiction medicine consultation when available
- All hospitalized persons with OUD should be offered medication for OUD as soon as possible
- Hospitals should provide harm reduction including education on sterile injection, provision of vaccination, and HIV PrEP
- Treating pain in persons with OUD is important to addiction and infection management
- Reducing stigma and rapidly responding to pain and withdrawal in hospitalized persons with OUD will promote retention in care

DISCLOSURE

EFE has received research support to UAB on her behalf from the National Institute of Health, Center for AIDS Research, Agency for Health Research and Quality (K12HS023009), the Gilead HIV Research Scholarship, Viiv, the Center for AIDS Research, the National Academy of Medicine.

REFERENCES

1. Wurcel AG, Anderson JE, Chui KK, et al. Increasing infectious endocarditis admissions among young people who inject drugs. Open Forum Infect Dis 2016; 3(3):ofw157.
2. Hsu DJ, McCarthy EP, Stevens JP, et al. Hospitalizations, costs and outcomes associated with heroin and prescription opioid overdoses in the United States 2001–12. Addiction 2017;112(9):1558–64.
3. Owens PL, Barrett ML, Weiss AJ, et al. Hospital inpatient utilization related to opioid overuse among adults, 1993–2012: statistical brief #177. Rockville (MD): Agency for Healthcare Research and Quality (US); 2006.
4. Mccarthy NL, Baggs J, See I, et al. Bacterial infections associated with substance use disorders, large cohort of United States Hospitals, 2012-2017. Clin Infect Dis 2020. https://doi.org/10.1093/cid/ciaa008.
5. Kasper KJ, Manoharan I, Hallam B, et al. A controlled-release oral opioid supports S. aureus survival in injection drug preparation equipment and may increase bacteremia and endocarditis risk. PLoS One 2019;14(8):e0219777.
6. Phillips KT, Stein MD. Risk practices associated with bacterial infections among injection drug users in Denver, Colorado. Am J Drug Alcohol Abuse 2010; 36(2):92–7.
7. Fink DS, Lindsay SP, Slymen DJ, et al. Abscess and self-treatment among injection drug users at four california syringe exchanges and their surrounding communities. Subst Use Misuse 2013;48(7):523–31.
8. Paquette CE, Syvertsen JL, Pollini RA. Stigma at every turn: Health services experiences among people who inject drugs. Int J Drug Policy 2018;57:104–10.
9. Summers PJ, Hellman JL, MacLean MR, et al. Negative experiences of pain and withdrawal create barriers to abscess care for people who inject heroin. A mixed methods analysis. Drug Alcohol Depend 2018;190:200–8.
10. Velez CM, Nicolaidis C, Korthuis PT, et al. "It's been an experience, a life learning experience": a qualitative study of hospitalized patients with substance use disorders. J Gen Intern Med 2017;32(3):296–303.
11. Parker CM, Hirsch JS, Hansen HB, et al. Facing opioids in the shadow of the HIV epidemic. N Engl J Med 2019;380(1):1–3.
12. National Institute on Drug Abuse. Medications to Treat Opioid Use Disorder 2020. Available at: https://www.drugabuse.gov/publications/research-reports/medications-to-treat-opioid-addiction/references. Accessed February 4, 2020.
13. Prevention CfDCa. New Data Show Growing Complexity of Drug Overdose Deaths in America. 2020. Available at: https://www.cdc.gov/media/releases/2018/p1221-complexity-drug-overdose.html.
14. Prevention CfDCa. U.S. State Prescribing Rates. 2017. Available at: https://www.cdc.gov/drugoverdose/maps/rxstate2017.html. Accessed February 4, 2020.
15. Project THCaU. HCUP Fast Stats- Opioid Hospital Use Map. Available at: https://www.hcup-us.ahrq.gov/faststats/OpioidUseMap?setting=IP. Accessed February 4, 2020.
16. Prevention CfDCa. Rural America in Crisis: The Changing Opioid Overdose Epidemic 2020. Available at: https://blogs.cdc.gov/publichealthmatters/2017/11/opioids/. Accessed February 4, 2020.
17. Collier MG, Doshani M, Asher A. Using population based hospitalization data to monitor increases in conditions causing morbidity among persons who inject drugs. J Community Health 2018. https://doi.org/10.1007/s10900-017-0458-9.

18. Fleischauer AT, Ruhl L, Rhea S, et al. Hospitalizations for endocarditis and associated health care costs among persons with diagnosed drug dependence - North Carolina, 2010-2015. MMWR Morb Mortal Wkly Rep 2017;66(22):569–73.
19. Eaton EF, Mathews RE, Lane PS, et al. A 9-point risk assessment for patients who inject drugs requiring intravenous antibiotics may allow health systems to focus inpatient resources on those at greatest risk of ongoing drug use. Clin Infect Dis 2018. https://doi.org/10.1093/cid/ciy722.
20. Rapoport AB, Fischer LS, Santibanez S, et al. Infectious diseases physicians' perspectives regarding injection drug use and related infections, United States, 2017. Open Forum Infect Dis 2018;5(7). https://doi.org/10.1093/ofid/ofy132.
21. Fanucchi LC, Lofwall MR, Nuzzo PA, et al. In-hospital illicit drug use, substance use disorders, and acceptance of residential treatment in a prospective pilot needs assessment of hospitalized adults with severe infections from injecting drugs. J Subst Abuse Treat 2018;92:64–9.
22. Rudasill SE, Sanaiha Y, Mardock AL, et al. Clinical outcomes of infective endocarditis in injection drug users. J Am Coll Cardiol 2019;73(5):559–70.
23. Wickersham JA, Azar MM, Cannon CM, et al. Validation of a brief measure of opioid dependence: the rapid opioid dependence screen (RODS). J Correct Health Care 2015;21(1):12–26.
24. Schuckit MA. Treatment of opioid-use disorders. N Engl J Med 2016;375(4): 357–68.
25. U.S. Department of Justice DEA. National Drug Threat Assessment 2018. 2018. Available at: https://www.dea.gov/sites/default/files/2018-11/DIR-032-18% 202018%20NDTA%20%5Bfinal%5D%20low%20resolution11-20.pdf. Accessed February 12, 2020.
26. Marks LR, Munigala S, Warren DK. Addiction medicine consultations reduce readmission rates for patients with serious infections from opioid use disorder. Clinical Infectious Diseases 2019;68(11):1935–7.
27. Botticelli MGM, Laderman M. Effective strategies for hospitals responding to the opioid crisis. Boston: Institute for Healthcare Improvement and The Grayken Center for Addiction at Boston Medical Center; 2019.
28. National Academies of Sciences E, Medicine. Opportunities to improve opioid use disorder and infectious disease services: integrating responses to a dual epidemic. Washington, DC: The National Academies Press; 2020. p. 220.
29. Administration SAaMHS. Number of DATA-waived Practitioners. Available at: https://www.samhsa.gov/medication-assisted-treatment/practitioner-program-data/certified-practitioners. Accessed December 28, 2019.
30. Rosenthal ES, Karchmer AW, Theisen-Toupal J, et al. Suboptimal addiction interventions for patients hospitalized with injection drug use-associated infective endocarditis. Am J Med 2016;129(5):481–5.
31. Jicha C, Saxon D, Lofwall MR, et al. Substance use disorder assessment, diagnosis, and management for patients hospitalized with severe infections due to injection drug use. J Addict Med 2019;13(1):69–74.
32. Wesson DR, Ling W. The clinical opiate withdrawal scale (COWS). J Psychoactive Drugs 2003;35(2):253–9.
33. Rodger L, Glockler-Lauf SD, Shojaei E, et al. Clinical characteristics and factors associated with mortality in first-episode infective endocarditis among persons who inject drugs. JAMA Netw open 2018;1(7):e185220.
34. Suzuki J. Medication-assisted treatment for hospitalized patients with intravenous-drug-use related infective endocarditis. Am J Addict 2016;25(3): 191–4.

35. Liebschutz JM, Crooks D, Herman D, et al. Buprenorphine treatment for hospital-ized, opioid-dependent patients: a randomized clinical trial. JAMA Intern Med 2014;174(8):1369–76.

36. D'Onofrio G, O'Connor PG, Pantalon MV, et al. Emergency department-initiated buprenorphine/naloxone treatment for opioid dependence: a randomized clinical trial. JAMA 2015;313(16):1636–44.

37. Englander H, Mahoney S, Brandt K, et al. Tools to support hospital-based addic-tion care: core components, values, and activities of the improving addiction care team. J Addict Med 2019;13(2):85–9.

38. Donroe JH, Holt SR, Tetrault JM. Caring for patients with opioid use disorder in the hospital. CMAJ 2016;188(17–18):1232–9.

39. Trowbridge P, Weinstein ZM, Kerensky T, et al. Addiction consultation services - Linking hospitalized patients to outpatient addiction treatment. J Subst Abuse Treat 2017;79:1–5.

40. Marks LR, Munigala S, Warren DK, et al. Addiction medicine consultations reduce readmission rates for patients with serious infections from opioid use disorder. Clin Infect Dis 2019;68(11):1935–7.

41. Theisen-Toupal J, Ronan MV, Moore A, et al. Inpatient management of opioid use disorder: a review for hospitalists. J Hosp Med 2017;12(5):369–74.

42. 8 Hour Online MAT Waiver Training. Available at: https://learning.pcssnow.org/p/ onlinematwaiver. Accessed January 25, 2020.

43. Special Circumstances for Providing Buprenorphine 2019. Available at: https://www. samhsa.gov/medication-assisted-treatment/legislation-regulations-guidelines/ special. Accessed May 22, 2019.

44. Special Circumstances for Providing Buprenorphine. Available at: https://www. samhsa.gov/medication-assisted-treatment/legislation-regulations-guidelines/ special. Accessed January 25, 2020.

45. Chan AC, Palepu A, Guh DP, et al. HIV-positive injection drug users who leave the hospital against medical advice: the mitigating role of methadone and social sup-port. J Acquir Immune Defic Syndr 2004;35(1):56–9.

46. Scheidegger C, Pietrzak J, Frei R. Disseminated candidiasis after intravenous use of oral methadone. Ann Intern Med 1991;115(7):576.

47. Gordon RJ, Lowy FD. Bacterial infections in drug users. N Engl J Med 2005; 353(18):1945–54.

48. Vlahov D, Sullivan M, Astemborski J, et al. Bacterial infections and skin cleaning prior to injection among intravenous drug users. Public Health Rep 1992;107(5): 595–8.

49. Binka M, Paintsil E, Patel A, et al. Disinfection of syringes contaminated with hep-atitis C virus by rinsing with household products. Open Forum Infect Dis 2015; 2(1):ofv017.

50. Raub JN, Vettese TE. Acute pain management in hospitalized adult patients with opioid dependence: a narrative review and guide for clinicians. J Hosp Med 2017;12(5):375–9.

51. Vlok R, An GH, Binks M, et al. Sublingual buprenorphine versus intravenous or intramuscular morphine in acute pain: A systematic review and meta-analysis of randomized control trials. Am J Emerg Med 2019;37(3):381–6.

52. McNeil R, Small W, Wood E, et al. Hospitals as a 'risk environment': an ethno-epidemiological study of voluntary and involuntary discharge from hospital against medical advice among people who inject drugs. Soc Sci Med 2014; 105:59–66.

53. Fanucchi L, Leedy N, Li J, et al. Perceptions and practices of physicians regarding outpatient parenteral antibiotic therapy in persons who inject drugs. J Hosp Med 2016;11(8):581–2.
54. Simon R, Snow R, Wakeman S. Understanding why patients with substance use disorders leave the hospital against medical advice: A qualitative study. Subst Abus 2019;1–7. https://doi.org/10.1080/08897077.2019.1671942.
55. Choi M, Kim H, Qian H, et al. Readmission rates of patients discharged against medical advice: a matched cohort study. PLoS One 2011;6(9):e24459.
56. Yong TY, Fok JS, Hakendorf P, et al. Characteristics and outcomes of discharges against medical advice among hospitalised patients. Intern Med J 2013;43(7): 798–802.
57. Seval N, Eaton E, Springer SA. Beyond antibiotics: a practical guide for the infectious disease physician to treat opioid use disorder in the setting of associated infectious diseases. Open Forum Infect Dis 2019. https://doi.org/10.1093/ofid/ofz539.

Outpatient Antimicrobial Treatment for People Who Inject Drugs

Hermione Hurley, MBChB, BE[a],*, Monica Sikka, MD[b],
Timothy Jenkins, MD, MSc[c], Evelyn Villacorta Cari, MD[d],
Alice Thornton, MD[d]

KEYWORDS

- Outpatient antimicrobial therapy • People who inject drugs, Skilled nursing facility

KEY POINTS

- People who inject substances have increasing rates of serious bacterial infections that require prolonged antibiotic treatment.
- Current models of care can create barriers to completion of treatment for people with substance use disorders.
- Successful programs reduce barriers, initiate and link patients to ongoing outpatient substance care, and offer patient-centered discharge options for completion of therapy.

BACKGROUND

People who inject substances have increasing rates of serious bacterial infections that require prolonged antibiotic treatment. Current models of care can create barriers to completion of treatment for people with substance use disorders (SUDs). Successful programs reduce barriers, initiate and link patients to ongoing outpatient substance care, and offer patient-centered discharge options for completion of antimicrobial therapy. This article reviews the changing epidemiology of infections associated with injection drug use, perceived barriers to care, features of successful programs, models of shared decision making at the time of discharge, and linkage to preventative care after antimicrobial completion.

[a] Center for Addiction Medicine, Denver Health and Hospital Authority, 667 Bannock Street, MC 3450, Denver, CO 80204, USA; [b] Division of Infectious Diseases, Oregon Health and Science University, 3181 Southwest Sam Jackson Park Road, L457, Portland, OR 97239, USA; [c] Division of Infectious Disease, Denver Health and Hospital Authority, 601 Broadway, MC4000, Denver, CO 80204, USA; [d] Division of Infectious Disease, University of Kentucky College of Medicine, 740 South Limestone, K512, Lexington, KY 40536-0284, USA
* Corresponding author.
E-mail address: hermione.hurley@dhha.org

Infect Dis Clin N Am 34 (2020) 525–538
https://doi.org/10.1016/j.idc.2020.06.009
id.theclinics.com

Epidemiology of Infectious Complications Associated with Injection Drug Use

As the opioid crisis has spread across the nation, the infectious complications associated with injection drug use have increased, including endocarditis, osteomyelitis, and skin and soft tissue infections.[1–3] A large retrospective study using data obtained from the Nationwide Inpatient Sample (NIS) reviewed hospitalizations related to opioid dependence and associated serious infections from 2002 to 2012. There was a significant increase in opioid-associated hospitalizations, from 3421 to 6535, during that time period. The distribution of cases based on diagnosis was endocarditis (46.4%), septic arthritis (29.8%), epidural abscess (16.6%), and osteomyelitis (7.4%).[1] In a literature review, Suzuki and colleagues[2,4,5] reported similar results, with the most common infections being bone and joint (37.9%; range, 0%–54%), endocarditis (21.0%; range, 0%–52%), skin and soft tissue (16.1%; range, 0%–36%), bacteremia (6.6%; range, 0%–53%), and abscess (5.0%; range, 0%–13%). A recent retrospective study of a large electronic health care database covering approximately 20% of US inpatient discharges showed that between 2012 and 2017, rates of infective endocarditis associated with SUDs increased from 19.9% to 39.4%, with smaller but significant increases seen in substance-related admissions for osteomyelitis, central nervous system abscesses, and skin soft tissue infections.[5]

Outpatient Antimicrobial Therapy is Uncommon for People Who Inject Drugs

For patients who not have a substance use disorder, prolonged antibiotic courses are typically completed with intravenous (IV) antibiotics that are self-administered through a central venous catheter in the outpatient setting, referred to as outpatient parenteral antibiotic therapy (OPAT). OPAT was initially described in the United States in 1974 for the management of chronic bronchopulmonary infections in patients with cystic fibrosis.[6] Since then, multiple studies have demonstrated that OPAT programs are a safe and cost-effective alternative to hospitalization for antimicrobial delivery in diverse populations with a variety of infections.[7] In 2018, the Infectious Diseases Society of America (IDSA) released an update of the Clinical Practice Guideline for the management of OPAT and strongly recommended that an infectious diseases (ID) consultation should be sought prior to the initiation of OPAT to lower the risk of hospital admission and provide "enhanced coordination of care after hospital discharge."[8,9]

However, many clinicians are reluctant to discharge people who inject drugs with a central venous catheter because of active substance use, frequent loss to follow-up, and complex psychosocial issues. The IDSA guidelines do not offer a definitive recommendation for this situation; they suggest that the decision should be made on a case-by-case basis.[8] Because of the severity and complexity of serious infections associated with injection drug use, the standard of care selected often involves hospitalization until completion of therapy. Patients are then relegated to inpatient treatment even after they are medically stable. It is common for patients with infections associated with injection drug use to have prolonged hospital stays. One southeastern hospital reported an average length of stay of 38 to 39.5 days for patients who were identified with an SUD and serious bacterial infection.[10,11] Prolonged admissions are costly to hospitals, unsatisfactory to patients and hospital personnel, and associated with low rates of treatment completion and significant risk of reinfection after discharge.[1,12]

The Negative Consequences of Prolonged Hospital Admission

Because of the significant limitations and barriers of existing outpatient antibiotic treatment options for people who inject drugs, clinicians frequently opt to keep patients in the hospital or another supervised medical facility to complete 4 to 6 weeks of IV antibiotic therapy.[13] The negative consequences for patients include feelings of isolation, challenges to retaining employment, financial stress, and inability to maintain family responsibilities. Notably, even in these monitored settings, rates of patient-reported, in-hospital substance use of up to 40% have been described,[10] and tampering with the central venous catheter, drug overdoses, and deaths occur.[10,14,15]

Intended antimicrobial courses are often not completed when the only offered treatment option is a prolonged hospital admission. People who inject drugs are among the patients most likely to have self-directed discharges (SDDs) or leave against medical advice (AMA), resulting in incomplete treatment of curable serious infections.[16] The rate of leaving prior to treatment completion in people who inject drugs has been reported to range from 11% to 30%.[10,17–19] Even when the treatment course is completed, only 20% to 50% of hospitalized people who inject drugs go on to engage in SUD treatment after discharge, and even fewer are retained in care.[20,21] Readmissions or emergency room visits are common for all people receiving OPAT, but have been found to be higher in all individuals who leave the hospital prior to treatment completion.[9,17] In 1 study, 30% of patients who left with SDD were readmitted within 30 days.[22]

In light of these major limitations, there is widespread dissatisfaction with current treatment options among clinicians.[13] Novel care models are urgently needed to facilitate safe and effective antibiotic therapy in this population after hospital discharge.

PERCEIVED BARRIERS TO OUTPATIENT TREATMENT

People who inject drugs have routinely been excluded from OPAT programs; thus, these patients often need to complete antimicrobial treatment in highly supervised settings.[4,23] A survey of ID physicians (n = 672) of the Emerging Infections Network revealed that most respondents (88%) reported treating at least 1 person who injects drugs monthly, with an injection drug use (IDU)-related infection.[13] Forty-one percent reported treating people who inject drugs with IDU-related infections on an inpatient unit for the entire course of antimicrobial treatment. Fanucchi and colleagues surveyed perception and practices of 66 physicians regarding the provision of OPAT for people who inject drugs. The largest barriers were socioeconomic factors (such as stable housing or transportation) and the clinician's concern for potential risk of patients misusing the central venous catheter. However, less than half of the respondents identified SUD treatment as essential to the OPAT decision.[23]

In published reports of OPAT for people who inject drugs, low rates of antibiotic treatment completion (52%)[24] and high rates of nonadherence to antibiotic doses (36%),[25] loss to follow up (47%), central venous catheter complications (7%),[15] and readmissions (16%–30%)[25,26] have been described as barriers to this treatment approach. In a retrospective study of 38 people who inject drugs who received OPAT for deep-seated infections, 23.7% were readmitted on at least 1 occasion during the study time frame.[27] This was more than double (10.1%) the overall admission rate for all OPAT patients in the study institution (**Box 1**).

However, multiple studies have reviewed various barriers to people who inject drugs receiving OPAT, and many of these concerns have been called into question. Fear of misuse of the peripherally inserted central catheter (PICC) line is a commonly reported clinician concern. However, this concern is not supported by literature, as this has been reported to occur in only to 0% to 2% of cases.[28–30] Another concern is whether patients will complete or adhere to OPAT. Although some studies have described low rates of completion, other recent studies have also shown that completion rates of OPAT have ranged from 72% to 100% for people who inject drugs with OPAT, rates comparable to those of other patients who receive OPAT.[15,27,29,31]

Box 1
Barriers to providing outpatient antimicrobial therapy for people who inject drugs

System Barriers[31,53]
- Facilities are often unwilling to provide outpatient intravenous treatment to PWID
- Few alternative treatment models (medical respite facilities, residential addiction centers)

Clinician Barriers[18,23,31]
- Lack of guidance for administration of OPAT programs in PWID
- Hesitance to initiate OPAT because of the potential for PICC misuse
- Fear of treatment nonadherence and subsequent reinfection
- Increased rates of OPAT complications compared with other populations
- Legal concerns

Patient Barriers[18,23,29,31]
- Active substance use
- Lack of engagement in mental health recovery services
- Lack of understanding about drug addiction and lack of motivation for treatment
- Presence of risk factors for relapse
- Previous history of SUD treatment failure
- Unsafe home environment
- Psychiatric comorbidities
- Inadequate social/family support
- Lack of insurance

Keeping a patient hospitalized for his or her antimicrobial therapy does not necessarily preclude the patient from using illicit drugs.[31] A small study of 42 people who inject drugs hospitalized with serious infections found that 17 (40.5%) of them had illicit drug use while hospitalized.[10] A small prospective study by the same authors found a trend toward less illicit drug use in people who inject drugs who received OPAT and buprenorphine versus those hospitalized without buprenorphine while on antimicrobials.[29]

Historically, hospitalized people who inject drugs have not been offered consistent treatment for their SUD. Two retrospective studies reviewed people who inject drugs hospitalized with serious infections at 2 academic centers and found less than optimal addiction interventions. Both studies reviewed discharge summaries to determine recommendations for medication-assisted treatment for people who inject drugs during hospitalization and after discharge. Although 1 study mentioned addiction in 55.9% of discharge summaries, only 7.8% of patients had a plan for SUD treatment upon discharge.[32] In the second study, 77.8% of discharge summaries documented SUD, yet only 7.4% mentioned pharmacotherapy for SUD, and no referrals or follow-ups for SUD were documented.[17]

Some programs have advocated and instituted addiction services to initiate medication for opioid use disorder (MOUD) in people who inject drugs hospitalized with serious infections. In a retrospective chart review of 125 hospitalized people who inject drugs or people with opioid use disorder (OUD), Marks and colleagues[24] found that addiction medicine consultation was associated with a greater rate of completion of antimicrobial therapy, fewer AMA discharges, and lower readmissions within 90 days of discharge.

FEATURES OF SUCCESSFUL OUTPATIENT TREATMENT

Successful OPAT for people who inject drugs shares some common characteristics of OPAT in the general population. A key component to a successful program should include an interdisciplinary team.[33] Most OPAT teams consist of the patient, physician or clinician, an infusion nurse, and a pharmacist. Some institutions also include a hospital case manager/social worker and family members or other caregivers[33] (**Box 2**).

A prospective observational study performed in Vancouver, Canada, established the necessity to provide a safe environment to improve patient treatment adherence using a 12-bed live-in street-based clinic.[34] This study compared 24 people who inject drugs versus 63 other patients who were prescribed OPAT. PICC line complications

---

Box 2
Features of successful outpatient programs for treatment completion

Institutional Support[33,36,48]
- Dedicated personnel time
- Staff education
- Financial support for patient engagement
- Support for interdisciplinary team
- Established program policies and procedures

Collaborative Teams[33,35,36,48,53]
- Dedicated multidisciplinary OPAT team
  ○ Infectious disease physician
  ○ Addiction specialist
  ○ Pharmacist
  ○ Nursing staff
  ○ Social work
  ○ Medical specialists as appropriate
- Vendor agreements with community partners (eg, home infusion, home health)
- Comprehensive discharge planning
- Frequent communication among team members/weekly team meetings
- Case management and wrap-around services
- Education of clinicians and team on workflow

Addiction Consultation[35,53]
- Assess substance use disorder
- Initiate MOUD if desired
- Provide patient education surrounding overdose prevention, harm reduction strategies (including naloxone rescue kit), and expected outcomes with MOUD
- Patient access to mental health recovery services

Discharge Planning[27,33–35]
- Assess safety of home environment
- Ensure reliable social support such as family or friends
- Discuss team expectations of patient while receiving OPAT
- Obtain signed patient consent/agreement
- Establish reliable means of contact between patient and interdisciplinary team
- Assessment of barriers to successful OPAT (eg, transportation, telephone access, and housing)
- Enroll patient in insurance and complete any required prior authorizations
- PICC education and counseling regarding risk

Outpatient Follow-Up[8,30,33,35,53]
- Establish guidelines for PICC removal
- Periodic PICC assessment for adulteration (some advocate tamper-evident access)
- Clinic follow-up appointments at predetermined intervals for accountability
- Continued assessment of active substance use, counseling, and treatment

Patient Role[27,28,35]
- Motivated and engaged in the process
- Increased distance from last drug use
- Reliable supportive network such as family or friends
- Prior abstinence or period of recovery

occurred in 11 of 24 people who inject drugs (46%) versus 15 of 63 other patients (24%), respectively. However, replacement of the line was only required in 3 of 24 people who inject drugs (13%) versus 9 of 63 other patients (14%), and 21 of 24 people who inject drugs (86%) versus 50 of 63 other patients (79%) completed treatments. A retrospective observational study compared 52 patients identified as people who inject drugs who were discharged home for OPAT (19%) or to skilled nursing facility (SNF)/rehabilitation (35%). Those who received OPAT at home did not have a significantly higher rate of complications compared with those who were discharged to an SNF/rehabilitation. However, patients discharged to SNF/rehabilitation had a higher rate of ongoing IDU (68%) than those discharged home (33%). Interestingly, patients discharged home had more documented SUD discharge planning (57%) than those discharged to SNF/rehabilitation (16%) and had higher rates of antibiotic course completion (81% vs 64%), respectively.[35]

Fanucchi and colleagues described an innovative care model that was the first randomized clinical trial of OPAT in hospitalized adults with OUD and serious injection-related infections. All patients enrolled received buprenorphine and IV antimicrobial therapy and were randomized to receive the treatment in the hospital (usual care control) versus at home (OPAT intervention).[29] Twenty patients were enrolled, and an important component of this study was that all participants received MOUD, started while inpatient and continued outpatient. A multidisciplinary team was involved: addiction medicine, ID consultant, OPAT nurse, social work, and mental health. There was a significant decrease in the average length of hospital stay (22.4 days vs 45.9 days), and all patients completed the recommended treatment. Unexpectedly, there were a greater proportion of urine samples negative for illicit opioids in the OPAT group compared with the hospitalized participants. In the discussion, the authors consider whether the ability to continue usual activities in a patient's own community improved treatment outcomes. Additionally, OPAT participants in the intervention arm expressed no desire to inject into their central venous catheter, and no participants reported catheter misuse in either group.[29]

ALTERNATIVES TO PROLONGED HOSPITALIZATION
Discharge with Central Venous Catheter to Home, Street, or Short-Stay Skilled Nursing Facility

A growing body of evidence suggests that OPAT may be feasible and safe in a select group of people who inject drugs with serious infections.[4] Enhanced coordination is essential to OPAT delivery in people who inject drugs. Available options include: home OPAT, short stay at an SNF, residential stay at a substance use treatment center, or use of medical respite facilities.[12,14,31] Management of serious infections in people who inject drugs with OPAT can be a challenge but is achievable.[15,29,36]

A retrospective study compared outcomes of people who inject drugs who received OPAT at home (n = 21) versus at an SNF/rehabilitation center (n = 31). Readmission rates were similar among patients who received OPAT at home (14%) versus those receiving OPAT at an SNF/rehabilitation center (29%).[35] Additionally, patients discharged home did not have a significantly higher rate of complications than those receiving care at an SNF/rehabilitation center (19% vs 35%, $P>.05$).[35]

Infusion Center for Daily Intravenous Antibiotics

An alternative approach to continue IV antibiotic therapy in the outpatient setting is for patients to come to an infusion center on a daily basis for antibiotics via a PICC. This has the advantage of sparing the need for and potential risks associated with a central venous catheter. However, daily venous access may be difficult or unacceptable to patients because of poor venous access. Furthermore, given concern with rates of nonadherence and loss to follow-up, there is a perceived risk that patients may not complete treatment and be at risk for severe adverse outcomes. To the authors' knowledge, there have been no studies of the effectiveness of daily infusion center visits for long-term antibiotic therapy in this population.

Intravenous Antibiotic Therapy During Intensive Residential Treatment

Several institutions have developed programs to treat people who inject drugs with serious bacterial infections with outpatient IV antibiotic therapy during intensive residential treatment. This allows patients to perform self-administered IV antibiotic therapy in a monitored setting while receiving comprehensive SUD treatment. Despite the potential benefits to patients and hospitals with this treatment approach, it requires substantial resources, and barriers such as low rates of eligibility and lack of patient interest in intensive residential treatment have limited its apparent utility. When feasible, this may be an excellent option for patients; however, this treatment approach is likely to meet the needs of only a select group of patients.

Long Half-Life Intravenous Antibiotics

Another approach to facilitate completion of antibiotic therapy in the outpatient setting involves the use of the long-acting lipoglycopeptides, dalbavancin, or oritavancin. These agents have a prolonged half-life and require only once-weekly infusion. Preliminary data suggest that 2 doses 1 week apart may be sufficient to treat bone and joint infections,[37] thus obviating the need for daily antibiotic therapy or a central venous catheter.[37] Although these agents are currently only approved by the US Food and Drug Administration for the treatment of skin and soft tissue infections, reports of off-label use for endovascular and other deep-seated infections in PWID have emerged.

In 1study, dalbavancin was used to treat 32 people who inject drugs hospitalized with serious *Staphylococcus aureus* infections including endocarditis, osteomyelitis, septic thrombophlebitis, spinal epidural infection, bacteremia, and septic arthritis.[38] After an initial period of daily IV antibiotic therapy, patients received between 1 and 5 doses of dalbavancin over several weeks. Most patients (56%) had a clinical response to treatment; however, 31% were lost to follow-up and had unevaluable outcomes. Other case series describing use of these agents have demonstrated low treatment completion rates (53%), frequent readmissions (18%–19%), and high rates of loss to follow-up (25%–47%).[38–40] This demonstrates that even with the advent of long-acting, once-weekly IV antibiotics, loss to follow-up is an important barrier to completion of antibiotic courses in this population. Moreover, these agents are costly, averaging about $4000 per dose. Before widespread use of these agents can be recommended, additional studies are needed to determine both their safety and efficacy for serious bacterial infections and their effectiveness in this patient population.

Oral Antibiotic Regimens

Recent landmark studies have demonstrated that oral antibiotics are as effective as IV antibiotics for endocarditis, osteomyelitis, and septic arthritis.[41–43] Although oral antibiotics are an attractive treatment option for PWID, clinicians are frequently hesitant to prescribe prolonged outpatient antibiotic courses to these patients out of concern for adverse clinical outcomes associated with failure to complete the antibiotic course[13] and the high rates of antibiotic nonadherence and loss to follow-up among people who inject drugs. Therefore, the generalizability of the recent oral antibiotic studies to the population of people who inject drugs is not clear. Indeed, only 5 (1.25%) patients in the trial of oral antibiotics for endocarditis[42] and no patients in the trial of oral antibiotics for bone and joint infection[43] were reported to use injection drugs. Studies of the clinical effectiveness of oral antibiotic regimens in this particular patient population are clearly warranted. It is likely that interventions to promote adherence to oral therapy and retention in care would be required for such an approach to be successful.

SHARED DECISION MAKING NEAR THE TIME OF DISCHARGE

Given the significant rates of noncompletion with exclusively prolonged hospitalization or home OPAT options, it is increasingly important to consider a patient-centered approach to treatment selection. One framework to create options for completion of antibiotic treatment outside of the hospital is by systematically reviewing specific risks and protective factors of SUD and OPAT in a multidisciplinary setting as part of discharge planning.[28] To augment the probability of completion of OPAT courses, patient preference should be considered and then options tailored to maximize the probability of successful treatment. Tools to review factors essential for safe OPAT courses have been described.[26,44] Discussion of risk and protective factors for outpatient treatment for people who inject drugs is critical to consider when considering options for treatment outside of the hospital (**Table 1**).

The goal of a meeting for discharge planning is to develop a safe and acceptable treatment plan for patients with SUD and serious infections requiring prolonged antimicrobials. A standardized approach to reviewing the following substance use history, patient goals and preferences, infection management, and antibiotic administration options can help create more treatment options for the patient.

Substance Use History

A comprehensive review of substance use including use practices and frequency, motivation for and stabilization on MOUD, social supports, and triggers for use can help determine if alternative therapies to in-hospital completion of antibiotics should be considered. Patients who have a more recent history of use, unstable use, or high-risk use are at increased risk of OPAT failure.[28] If a patient is interested in MOUD, initiation while in the hospital should be strongly considered.[36,45] Identifying if a central venous catheter may be a trigger for substance use allows clinicians to consider risks of antibiotic delivery methods and tailor antibiotic route and setting. There are tools to perform a systematic assessment of the safety of central venous catheters in the community by reviewing cognitive factors, substance use triggers, and social supports.[44] The assessed risk of having a line in patients may steer a clinician toward alternative treatment options such as oral antibiotics or long-acting agents at hospital discharge or at an infusion center. If a central venous catheter in the community is deemed safe, the patient may be offered home infusion or therapy at an infusion center.

Patient Goals and Preferences

Consideration of patient's goals and preferences including desired discharge location or desired means of engagement with SUD care can help create more patient-acceptable treatment options. It is critical to be transparent with the patient about his or her infection and possible progression of infection with inadequate or partial treatment. Only then can patient preferences and goals be seriously considered along with the ID and SUD factors to provide alternative therapy recommendations. Respecting a patient's desire to go home to family, to address his or her SUD, or to

Table 1 Discharge planning decision matrix			
Possible treatment options	IV antibiotics in the hospital with inpatient addiction care	Long-acting injectable or oral antibiotics with linkage to outpatient SUD care	IV antibiotics at home or infusion center with harm reduction
	IV antibiotics at SNF with linkage to outpatient SUD care	IV antibiotics at home or at an infusion center with linkage to outpatient SUD care	Long-acting injectable or oral antibiotics with harm reduction

Goal: Safe, acceptable treatment plan for PWID with serious infections requiring prolonged antibiotics.

Substance use considerations - Infection management options (type of infection, therapeutic options).

Patient goals and preferences - Antibiotic administration options (route and location).

stay in the hospital may lead to increased rates of adherence to therapy and thus decrease discharges prior to treatment completion. A discharge planning meeting can also provide a venue to explore options to assist with housing insecurity or desires for substance treatment by providing linkage to programs that can assist long term in housing options and community SUD programs.

Infection Management

A review of infection type, modalities for antimicrobial treatment, and access to follow-up with the primary care provider (PCP) or specialty clinician should be performed. Having a PCP can be protective[46,47] for readmission during OPAT, and ID teams may have more confidence to explore out-of-hospital treatment plans for patients who have an established PCP or who will be scheduled with one once discharged. Respecting patient's wishes that involve nonstandard of care antibiotic therapy may not be the most preferred option from the clinician's standpoint, but completing therapy may be better than the alternative of no therapy or partial therapy.

Antibiotic Administration Options

To determine options for antibiotic administration, the location and route that are deemed safe and feasible for a patient to receive antibiotics must be considered. Factors that contribute to making this determination include insurance coverage, means of communication, the living environment, and perceived risk of central venous catheter in the community. Case managers are essential to elucidating insurance coverage, which dictates what outpatient options are feasible, such as SNF, home infusion, or infusion center. If a patient's insurance coverage does not have a transportation benefit, completing therapy at an infusion center may not be a viable option. In this instance, an SNF or in-hospital stay may be preferred. A systematic review of a patient's living environment may reveal housing insecurity or a home without running water or refrigeration, thus eliminating home infusion as an option. Alternatively, if such a review reveals that a patient has supportive family and stable housing, OPAT with home infusion may be considered. Reliable means of communication is important, as it is essential that home health companies or home infusion centers are able to contact the patient. Some OPAT teams require 2 or more working telephone numbers as points of contact.[27,48] Access to a telephone also allows for follow-up appointment scheduling and reminders and increases the patient's ability to report adverse effects of medications or concerns.

In summary, an individualized review of these four factors as part of discharge planning can help expand treatment options beyond a prolonged inpatient stay and allows evaluation of treatment feasible and acceptable to patients and clinicians.

LINKAGE TO PREVENTATIVE AND SUBSTANCE USE CARE

Patient care does not stop with the completion of antimicrobials. Successful holistic care requires assistance to enroll for insurance, continued substance use treatment, engagement with the PCP, and the offer of preventative care. People with SUDs often experience shame and judgment when interacting with health care systems. The successful completion and resolution of a serious infection offer a window of opportunity to engage in productive ways with health care. Preventative care should be offered to reduce the chance of reinfection or new infection. Preventive care includes harm reduction activities like discussion of local syringe services programs, advocacy for safe injection sites, early access to wound care, and provision of naloxone prescriptions in case of overdose. Vaccination for hepatitis A, hepatitis B, influenza, tetanus, diphtheria, and pertussis can reduce the chance of avoidable morbidity.[49–51] Screening and linkage to treatment for hepatitis C virus and human immunodeficiency virus (HIV) infection will improve individual outcomes and reduce community transmission.[52] At institutions with the ability to colocate substance and ID care, this approach may create a point of contact to offer low-barrier care such as screening for sexually transmitted infections, contraception, and pre-exposure prophylaxis (PrEP) for HIV.

DISCUSSION

Treatment of serious infections for people who inject drugs can be challenging. But as discussed, the current binary model of prolonged hospitalization or home OPAT does not assure treatment completion or remove the risk of complications. It is recognized that providing outpatient completion of antimicrobial treatment for people with SUDs is labor intensive, but prolonged hospitalizations are costly, often unsatisfactory to patients, and can lead to increased discharge prior to completion of therapy. There are no convincing data that inpatient stays are superior to OPAT in people with SUDs. In the search for patient-centered care associated with a rising epidemic, one must continue to strive for novel collaborative approaches to ensure that each person is treated in the best way possible to successfully complete antimicrobial therapy, and then linked to a path of lifelong health care.

FINANCIAL DISCLOSURES AND CONFLICTS OF INTEREST

H. Hurley provides waiver training courses for clinicians to become buprenorphine prescribers through the Providers Clinical Support System. M. Sikka has no financial disclosures or conflicts of interest to report. E.V. Cari has no financial disclosures or conflicts of interest to report. T. Jenkins has no financial disclosures or conflicts of interest to report. A. Thornton serves as clinical consultant, Diagnostic Compliance Site Visit, Health Resources and Service Administration, HIV AIDS Bureau for Community Based Programs Ryan White HIV Clinics Part C/D (2002–2020). PON2 729 1900003238 Thornton (PI) 09/30/2018-09/29/2021 KORE-WRAP KY Cabinet for Health and Family Services. Integrating Medication Assisted Treatment for Opioid Use Disorder with Infectious Disease Care Wrap Around Services.

REFERENCES

1. Ronan MV, Herzig SJ. Hospitalizations related to opioid abuse/dependence and associated serious infections increased sharply, 2002-12. Health Aff (Millwood) 2016;35(5):832–7.
2. Wurcel AG, Anderson JE, Chui KK, et al. Increasing infectious endocarditis admissions among young people who inject drugs. Open Forum Infect Dis 2016; 3(3):ofw157.
3. Jackson KA, Bohm MK, Brooks JT, et al. Invasive methicillin-resistant staphylococcus aureus infections among persons who inject drugs - six sites, 2005-2016. MMWR Morb Mortal Wkly Rep 2018;67(22):625–8.
4. Suzuki J, Johnson J, Montgomery M, et al. Outpatient parenteral antimicrobial therapy among people who inject drugs: a review of the literature. Open Forum Infect Dis 2018;5(9):ofy194.
5. McCarthy NL, Baggs J, See I, et al. Bacterial infections associated with substance use disorders, large cohort of United States Hospitals, 2012-2017. Clin Infect Dis 2020. https://doi.org/10.1093/cid/ciaa008.
6. Rucker RW, Harrison GM. Outpatient intravenous medications in the management of cystic fibrosis. Pediatrics 1974;54(3):358–60.
7. Williams DN, Baker CA, Kind AC, et al. The history and evolution of outpatient parenteral antibiotic therapy (OPAT). Int J Antimicrob Agents 2015;46(3):307–12.
8. Norris AH, Shrestha NK, Allison GM, et al. 2018 Infectious Diseases Society of America clinical practice guideline for the management of outpatient parenteral antimicrobial therapy. Clin Infect Dis 2019;68(1):e1–35.
9. Keller SC, Ciuffetelli D, Bilker W, et al. The impact of an infectious diseases transition service on the care of outpatients on parenteral antimicrobial therapy. J Pharm Technol 2013;29(5):205–14.
10. Fanucchi LC, Lofwall MR, Nuzzo PA, et al. In-hospital illicit drug use, substance use disorders, and acceptance of residential treatment in a prospective pilot needs assessment of hospitalized adults with severe infections from injecting drugs. J Subst Abuse Treat 2018;92:64–9.
11. Gundelly P, Burgess DS, Boulay J, et al. 921: Prevalence of hepatitis C infection and epidemiology of infective endocarditis in intravenous drug users in central Kentucky. Open Forum Infect Dis 2014;1(S266).
12. Jafari S, Joe R, Elliot D, et al. A community care model of intravenous antibiotic therapy for injection drug users with deep tissue infection for "reduce leaving against medical advice.". Int J Ment Health Addict 2015;13:49–58.
13. Rapoport AB, Fischer LS, Santibanez S, et al. Infectious diseases physicians' perspectives regarding injection drug use and related infections, United States, 2017. Open Forum Infect Dis 2018;5(7):ofy132.
14. Beieler A, Magaret A, Zhou Y, et al. Outpatient parenteral antimicrobial therapy in vulnerable populations– people who inject drugs and the homeless. J Hosp Med 2019;14(2):105–9.
15. Dobson PM, Loewenthal MR, Schneider K, et al. Comparing injecting drug users with others receiving outpatient parenteral antibiotic therapy. Open Forum Infect Dis 2017;4(4):ofx183.
16. McNeil R, Small W, Wood E, et al. Hospitals as a 'risk environment': an ethnoepidemiological study of voluntary and involuntary discharge from hospital against medical advice among people who inject drugs. Soc Sci Med 2014; 105:59–66.

17. Jicha C, Saxon D, Lofwall MR, et al. Substance use disorder assessment, diagnosis, and management for patients hospitalized with severe infections due to injection drug use. J Addict Med 2019;13(1):69–74.
18. Mertz D, Viktorin N, Wolbers M, et al. Appropriateness of antibiotic treatment in intravenous drug users, a retrospective analysis. BMC Infect Dis 2008;8:42.
19. Ti L, Ti L. Leaving the hospital against medical advice among people who use illicit drugs: a systematic review. Am J Public Health 2015;105(12):e53–9.
20. Trowbridge P, Weinstein ZM, Kerensky T, et al. Addiction consultation services - Linking hospitalized patients to outpatient addiction treatment. J Subst Abuse Treat 2017;79:1–5.
21. Naeger S, Mutter R, Ali MM, et al. Post-discharge treatment engagement among patients with an opioid-use disorder. J Subst Abuse Treat 2016;69:64–71.
22. Choi M, Kim H, Qian H, et al. Readmission rates of patients discharged against medical advice: a matched cohort study. PLoS One 2011;6(9):e24459.
23. Fanucchi L, Leedy N, Li J, et al. Perceptions and practices of physicians regarding outpatient parenteral antibiotic therapy in persons who inject drugs. J Hosp Med 2016;11(8):581–2.
24. Marks LR, Munigala S, Warren DK, et al. Addiction medicine consultations reduce readmission rates for patients with serious infections from opioid use disorder. Clin Infect Dis 2019;68(11):1935–7.
25. Beieler AM, Dellit TH, Chan JD, et al. Successful implementation of outpatient parenteral antimicrobial therapy at a medical respite facility for homeless patients. J Hosp Med 2016;11(8):531–5.
26. Eaton EF, Mathews RE, Lane PS, et al. A 9-point risk assessment for patients who inject drugs and require intravenous antibiotics: focusing inpatient resources on patients at greatest risk of ongoing drug use. Clin Infect Dis 2019;68(6):1041–3.
27. O'Callaghan K, Tapp S, Hajkowicz K, et al. Outcomes of patients with a history of injecting drug use and receipt of outpatient antimicrobial therapy. Eur J Clin Microbiol Infect Dis 2019;38(3):575–80.
28. Buehrle DJ, Shields RK, Shah N, et al. Risk factors associated with outpatient parenteral antibiotic therapy program failure among intravenous drug users. Open Forum Infect Dis 2017;4(3):ofx102.
29. Fanucchi LC, Walsh SL, Thornton AC, et al. Outpatient parenteral antimicrobial therapy plus buprenorphine for opioid use disorder and severe injection-related infections. Clin Infect Dis 2020;70(6):1226–9.
30. Ho J, Archuleta S, Sulaiman Z, et al. Safe and successful treatment of intravenous drug users with a peripherally inserted central catheter in an outpatient parenteral antibiotic treatment service. J Antimicrob Chemother 2010;65(12):2641–4.
31. Camsari UM, Libertin CR. Small-town America's despair: infected substance users needing outpatient parenteral therapy and risk stratification. Cureus 2017;9(8):e1579.
32. Rosenthal ES, Karchmer AW, Theisen-Toupal J, et al. Suboptimal addiction interventions for patients hospitalized with injection drug use-associated infective endocarditis. Am J Med 2016;129(5):481–5.
33. Tice AD, Rehm SJ, Dalovisio JR, et al. Practice guidelines for outpatient parenteral antimicrobial therapy. IDSA guidelines. Clin Infect Dis 2004;38(12):1651–72.
34. Hill A, WA, Marsh D, et al. Pilot assessment of intravenous antibiotic therapy in a live-in street-based clinic, for infections in intravenous drug users (IVDU's). 2006. Available at: https://idsaconfexcom/idsa/2006/webprogram/Paper22373html. Accessed January 27, 2020.

35. D'Couto HT, Robbins GK, Ard KL, et al. Outcomes according to discharge location for persons who inject drugs receiving outpatient parenteral antimicrobial therapy. Open Forum Infect Dis 2018;5(5):ofy056.

36. Englander H, Wilson T, Collins D, et al. Lessons learned from the implementation of a medically enhanced residential treatment (MERT) model integrating intravenous antibiotics and residential addiction treatment. Subst Abus 2018;39(2): 225–32.

37. Morata L, Cobo J, Fernandez-Sampedro M, et al. Safety and efficacy of prolonged use of dalbavancin in bone and joint infections. Antimicrob Agents Chemother 2019;63(5):e02280.

38. Bryson-Cahn C, Beieler AM, Chan JD, et al. Dalbavancin as secondary therapy for serious staphylococcus aureus infections in a vulnerable patient population. Open Forum Infect Dis 2019;6(2):ofz028.

39. Bork JT, Heil EL, Berry S, et al. Dalbavancin use in vulnerable patients receiving outpatient parenteral antibiotic therapy for invasive gram-positive infections. Infect Dis Ther 2019;8(2):171–84.

40. Morrisette T, Miller MA, Montague BT, et al. Long-acting lipoglycopeptides: "lineless antibiotics" for serious infections in persons who use drugs. Open Forum Infect Dis 2019;6(7):ofz274.

41. Bundgaard H, Ihlemann N, Gill SU, et al. Long-term outcomes of partial oral treatment of endocarditis. N Engl J Med 2019;380(14):1373–4.

42. Iversen K, Ihlemann N, Gill SU, et al. Partial oral versus intravenous antibiotic treatment of endocarditis. N Engl J Med 2019;380(5):415–24.

43. Li HK, Rombach I, Zambellas R, et al. Oral versus intravenous antibiotics for bone and joint infection. N Engl J Med 2019;380(5):425–36.

44. Englander H, Mahoney S, Brandt K, et al. Tools to support hospital-based addiction care: core components, values, and activities of the improving addiction care team. J Addict Med 2019;13(2):85–9.

45. Englander H, Weimer M, Solotaroff R, et al. Planning and designing the improving addiction care team (IMPACT) for hospitalized adults with substance use disorder. J Hosp Med 2017;12(5):339–42.

46. Felder KK, Marshall LM, Vaz LE, et al. Risk factors for complications during outpatient parenteral antimicrobial therapy for adult orthopedic and neurosurgical infections. South Med J 2016;109(1):53–60.

47. Means L, Bleasdale S, Sikka M, et al. Predictors of hospital readmission in patients receiving outpatient parenteral antimicrobial therapy. Pharmacotherapy 2016;36(8):934–9.

48. Thornton AC. Optimizing outcomes through multi-disciplinary inpatient teams: lessons from Kentucky. IDWEEK 2019 Wash DC, Oct 3, 2019. 2019.

49. Springer SA, Korthuis PT, Del Rio C. Integrating treatment at the intersection of opioid use disorder and infectious disease epidemics in medical settings: a call for action after a National Academies of Sciences, Engineering, and Medicine Workshop. Ann Intern Med 2018;169(5):335–6.

50. Thakarar K, Weinstein ZM, Walley AY. Optimising health and safety of people who inject drugs during transition from acute to outpatient care: narrative review with clinical checklist. Postgrad Med J 2016;92(1088):356–63.

51. Peak CM, Stous SS, Healy JM, et al. Homelessness and hepatitis A - San Diego County, 2016-2018. Clin Infect Dis 2019. https://doi.org/10.1093/cid/ciz788.

52. MacArthur GJ, van Velzen E, Palmateer N, et al. Interventions to prevent HIV and hepatitis C in people who inject drugs: a review of reviews to assess evidence of effectiveness. Int J Drug Policy 2014;25(1):34–52.
53. Fanucchi LC, Walsh SL, Thornton AC, et al. Integrated outpatient treatment of opioid use disorder and injection-related infections: a description of a new care model. Prev Med 2019;128:105760.

Applying the Infectious Diseases Literature to People who Inject Drugs

David P. Serota, MD, MSc[a],*, Teresa A. Chueng, MD, MPH[a,b],
Marcos C. Schechter, MD[c]

KEYWORDS

- Opioid use disorder • Injection drug use • Endocarditis • Antibacterials
- Outpatient parenteral antimicrobial therapy • Osteomyelitis • Harm reduction

KEY POINTS

- Application of the existing infectious disease (ID) literature to people who inject drugs (PWID) must consider their unique medical, psychological, and social challenges.
- Outpatient parenteral antimicrobial therapy can be successful among select PWID with injection drug use-associated (IDU) infections, especially when the alternative is prolonged hospitalization for intravenous antibiotics.
- Data supporting the use of oral antibiotics for severe bacterial infections should be applied with caution to PWID, and close ID follow-up and consideration of barriers to adherence to oral antibiotics are required.
- Literature on surgical management of IDU-associated endocarditis suggests worse long-term outcomes compared with other causes of endocarditis, but there are no prospective data comparing medical versus surgical approaches for IDU-associated endocarditis and little information on the effect of addiction treatment.

INTRODUCTION

Increasing rates of opioid use disorder have resulted in an epidemic of infectious complications of injection drug use (IDU). This includes outbreaks of human immunodeficiency virus (HIV)[1] and hepatitis C virus (HCV),[2] as well as increasing hospitalizations from skin and soft tissue infections (SSTIs), osteomyelitis, septic arthritis, bacteremia, central nervous system infections, and endocarditis.[3–7] Despite increasing incidence

a Division of Infectious Diseases, Department of Medicine, University of Miami Miller School of Medicine, 1120 Northwest 14 Street, Suite 851, Miami, FL 33136, USA; b Jackson Memorial Hospital, Jackson Health System, Miami, FL, USA; c Division of Infectious Diseases, Department of Medicine, Emory University, 49 Jesse Hill Jr Dr SE, Atlanta, GA 30303, USA
* Corresponding author.
E-mail address: dserota@med.miami.edu
Twitter: @serotavirus (D.P.S.); @teresachueng (T.A.C.); @limbsandlungs (M.C.S.)

Infect Dis Clin N Am 34 (2020) 539–558
https://doi.org/10.1016/j.idc.2020.06.010
0891-5520/20/© 2020 Elsevier Inc. All rights reserved.

id.theclinics.com

of IDU-associated infectious diseases, the best approach to management is unclear, varies widely, and remains understudied.[8-10] There is a critical need to identify the best ways to care for patients with IDU-associated infections.

To answer questions about the treatment of patients with IDU-associated infections, clinicians are tasked with applying the best available evidence, yet this research has often excluded people who inject drugs (PWID). Over the past few years, the literature has provided some answers to many of the fundamental questions in infectious diseases (IDs). With increased interest in evidence-based medicine, funding for pragmatic clinical trials, and democratization of the medical literature through social media, many long-held dogmas have been reversed based on robust clinical data. Examples include studies showing noninferiority of oral versus intravenous (IV) antibiotics for certain severe infections,[11,12] shorter versus longer courses of antibiotics,[13] and bactericidal versus bacteriostatic antibiotics.[14] Care must be taken when applying the ID literature to PWID. In this article, the authors will first describe important differences between PWID and the general population represented in clinical trials. Next, they propose an approach to using the literature to inform the management of IDU-associated infections. The authors then apply these principles to important evidence-based practices and provide a framework for designing effective treatment plans for PWID with severe infections.

DIFFERENCES BETWEEN PEOPLE WHO INJECT DRUGS AND PATIENTS REPRESENTED IN CLINICAL TRIALS

Recognizing differences between PWID and patients typically represented in clinical trials is important to appropriately contextualize these data for patients with IDU-associated infections. **Table 1** describes unique attributes of PWID and implications of how these differences from the general population may affect infection-related outcomes. **Table 2** presents common drug-drug interactions relevant to PWID presenting with IDU-associated infections.

APPLYING EVIDENCE-BASED PRACTICES TO INJECTION DRUG USE-ASSOCIATED INFECTIONS

In order to apply the ID literature to PWID, the authors suggest answering 3 questions about each evidence-based practice considered:

What is the evidence for this practice in the general population?
What is the evidence for this practice specifically among PWID?
What are the risks, benefits, and implications for applying this practice to PWID?

The focus of this article is on management questions in the treatment of severe IDU-associated infections requiring hospitalization (**Table 3**). The purpose of this article is not to provide a comprehensive guide to the management of all IDU-associated infections, but rather to build a framework for applying the best available evidence to a vulnerable population in a thoughtful and informed manner.

OUTPATIENT PARENTERAL ANTIMICROBIAL THERAPY FOR INJECTION DRUG USE-ASSOCIATED INFECTIONS
Evidence for Outpatient Parenteral Antimicrobial Therapy in the General Population

Outpatient parenteral antimicrobial therapy (OPAT) allows patients to receive IV antimicrobials outside of the acute care hospital setting. Patients receiving OPAT usually require placement of a peripherally inserted central catheter (PICC) to facilitate

Table 1
How people who inject drugs differ from the general population represented in clinical trials for management of severe infections

Characteristics of People Who Inject Drugs	Implications for Injection Drug Use-Associated Infections
Younger age and fewer comorbidities • Median age of IDU-endocarditis patients almost half that of non-IDU-associated endocarditis (33 vs 63 y)[79]	• More physiologic reserve to survive severe infections than older multimorbid patients[80,81] • Less likely to experience life-threatening adverse events from antimicrobials[82,83] • May be able to tolerate longer courses of riskier antimicrobials (such as trimethoprim-sulfamethoxazole)
More mental health disorders • 29% with depression, 22% have attempted suicide, and symptoms of post-traumatic stress disorder are common[84] • Higher prevalence of substance-induced mood disorders, personality disorders, and anxiety disorders[85,86]	• Barriers to adhere to medical treatment plans • Drug interactions between psychoactive medications, illicit drugs, and antimicrobials
More chronic viral infections • Among PWID, global HIV prevalence is 18%, and in the United States it is 7%[87,88] • More than 50% of PWID are antibody-positive for HCV and 9% have chronic hepatitis B virus infection[88]	• Immunodeficiency of advanced HIV increases the chances of both opportunistic and typical infections, as does chronic liver disease from HCV or HBV • Drug interactions between antiretroviral therapy (ART) and antimicrobials often used for the treatment of severe infections
Stigmatization by health care system • Many report experiences of dehumanization and discrimination[89] • Experiences of trauma during prolonged hospitalization[28]	• Associated with delay in presenting for health care, self-treatment attempts, and seeking informal therapies from nonmedical personnel[90,91] • Untreated withdrawal and undertreated pain fuel behaviors like leaving the hospital AMA (or early discharge) and in-hospital illicit drug use[92,93] • Stigmatization of drug use may lead PWID to present with more advanced disease, creates barriers to completing care plans, and often results in early discharge without antimicrobials or follow-up[30]
More social barriers to care • 60% report past-year homelessness[94] • 74% uninsured, and 19% did not seek care from a medical provider within the last year[95]	• Difficulty adhering to medical treatment plans while homeless • Lack of access to follow-up medical care and difficulty paying for medications

antimicrobial infusions, either at home, in a skilled nursing facility (SNF), nursing home, or other institution. OPAT has been deemed safe and effective for a variety of severe infections, including endocarditis.[15,16] The 2018 Infectious Diseases Society of America OPAT guidelines enumerate the benefits of OPAT, which include decreased hospital lengths of stay, reduced health care costs, fewer hospital acquired infections, and increased patient satisfaction, when compared with completing hospital-based antimicrobial therapy (HBAT).[15] Yet, although there are definite benefits to OPAT overall, the harms have been less well-defined.[17] For one of the most common OPAT

Table 2
Common drug interactions between antimicrobials and medications for opioid use disorder

Antibiotic Class	Concern	Antibiotic	Medication for Opioid Use Disorder		
			Methadone	Buprenorphine	XR-Naltrexone
Fluoroquinolones	QTc prolongation – risk for adverse CV events increased with structural heart disease, electrolyte disorders, and likely by use of multiple QTc prolonging agents (eg,: SSRI)[96–100]	Moxifloxacin – highest QTc effect and strongest association with CV events among FQs[101] Levofloxacin – lower QTc effect and association with CV events compared with moxifloxacin[101] Ciprofloxacin – lower QTc effect and association with CV events compared with moxifloxacin and levofloxacin[101] Delafloxacin – industry-sponsored studies suggest no QTc effect; limited postmarketing data[108,109]	Associated with QTc prolongation, but weak association with CV events Most cases reported to the FDA had other risk factors for QTc prolongation[102–104]	In vitro blockage of cardiac potassium voltage-gated channels, but no QTc prolongation in the absence of concomitant CYP inhibitors[105–107]	Not associated with QTc prolongation

	serotonin toxicity – risk for	Linezolid – MAOI	Weak serotonin reuptake inhibitor	No serotonin reuptake inhibitor activity predicted in vitro[114]	Not associated with serotonin toxicity
Oxazolidinones	serotonin toxicity increased by use of >1 serotonergic agent (eg, SSRI, MDMA, cocaine)	Most linezolid-associated serotonin toxicity cases reported were also on an SSRI[110] One case control study showed similar risk for serotonin toxicity when linezolid is used with or without an SSRI[111] Tedizolid – preclinical studies suggest less MAOI compared with linezolid and lower risk for serotonin toxicity Patients on SSRI excluded from clinical trials[116] Limited postmarketing data	One case report of serotonin toxicity associated with methadone and linezolid coadministration[112] Package insert recommends careful observation with slow incremental methadone doses if used together with an MAOI or ≤14 d of stopping a MAOI[113]	One published report of serotonin toxicity in patient taking tricyclic antidepressants Prescribing information does not recommend use together with an MAOI or ≤14 d of stopping a MAOI[115]	
Rifamycins	CYP induction leading to increased metabolism of CYP substrates Induction can occur within hours of first dose Induction reversal can take up to 2 weeks after discontinuation	Rifampin – potent CYP3A inhibitor Rifabutin – less potent CYP3A inhibitor compared with rifampin Limited clinical data for bacterial infections compared with rifampin[120]	Methadone is a CYP substrate and rifampin-induced withdrawal is well described.[117] Rifabutin does not appear to precipitate methadone withdrawal. Rifamycin/methadone combination not contraindicated, but careful monitoring needed[118]	Buprenorphine is a CYP substrate, and rifampin coadministration can induce withdrawal Rifabutin decreases buprenorphine levels, but does not appear to precipitate withdrawal Buprenorphine decreases rifabutin levels, but clinical significance unclear[119] Rifamycin/buprenorphine combination not contraindicated, but careful monitoring needed Consider rifabutin therapeutic drug monitoring	Not metabolized by CYPs No known interaction with rifamycins

Abbreviations: CV, cardiovascular; FQ, fluoroquinolone; MAOI, monoamine oxidase inhibitor; MDMA, 3,4-methylenedioxymethamphetamine (ecstasy); SSRI, selective serotonin reuptake inhibitor.

Table 3
Benefits and risks of implementing selected evidence-based practices for injection drug use-associated infections

	Benefits	Risks
OPAT vs extended hospitalization	• Completing treatment in more acceptable environment • Increased autonomy, ability to reintegrate, and enter recovery • Avoid traumatic aspects of extended hospitalization	• Nonadherence with potential for worsening infection • PICC-associated complications • Lack of close monitoring for toxicity and worsening infection • Exposure to drug use triggers
Oral vs intravenous antibiotics	• Helps avoid prolonged hospitalization • Increased autonomy, ability to reintegrate, and enter recovery • Lack of need for PICC • Allows most diverse discharge options	• Nonadherence with potential for worsening infection • Less clinical experience and data for PWID • Lack of close monitoring for toxicity and worsening infection • Exposure to drug use triggers • Requires close outpatient follow-up that may not be feasible • More drug-drug interactions
Shorter vs longer course antibiotics	• Less risk for antibiotic adverse events • Potential for shorter hospitalization and need for IV antibiotics	• Requires close outpatient follow up for response to treatment • Little clinical data specific to PWID
Long-acting IV vs standard oral or IV antibiotics	• IV bioavailability without the need to remain hospitalized • No need for PICC • Given long half-life, may be more tolerant of nonadherence	• High cost • Logistical difficulties of finding infusion chair • Only for gram-positive organisms
Surgery vs medical management	• Decreased complications/tissue destruction by infection (eg, shortened duration of sepsis, fewer debilitating emboli) • Potential for shorter course antibiotics, and shorter hospitalization	• Increased risk of reinfection, prosthetic device infection, especially in setting of ongoing drug use • Finite lifespan of many prosthetic devices

indications, *Staphylococcus aureus* bacteremia, Townsend and colleagues[18] documented an adverse event rate of 33% and 90-day readmission rate of 64% among patients receiving OPAT; however, there was no comparison to a group receiving HBAT. OPAT has become standard of care for most infections requiring an extended period of IV antimicrobials, and it is supported by strong evidence.

Evidence for Outpatient Parenteral Antimicrobial Therapy Among People Who Inject Drugs

Guidelines do not explicitly make a recommendation for or against providing OPAT to PWID, but recommend evaluation on a case-by-case basis.[15] However, many individual OPAT programs, home infusion companies, and hospitals have guidelines prohibiting OPAT for patients with a history of substance use disorders (SUDs) and PWID in particular.[9,10,19] Suzuki and colleagues[20] performed a review of published OPAT cohorts including PWID. Successful completion of OPAT ranged from 72% to 100% among studies reporting this outcome. Among studies that directly compared PWID versus OPAT among other patients, differences in treatment failure, readmission, mortality, and reinfection rates were negligible. PICC complications ranged from 3% to 9% across the cohorts, although some programs utilized special tamper-proof devices and frequent nurse oversight that might not be standard of care or available in most OPAT programs. Among studies comparing PICC complications between PWID and other patients, there were no significant differences. Patients were discharged to a mix of home, SNF, medical respite programs, and substance use rehabilitation programs. Home OPAT had no worse outcomes than those completing OPAT in an SNF, and patients have far better experiences with home OPAT versus SNF.[21,22]

There is reason to believe that treatment of the underlying SUD, especially in the case of OUD, has major implications for the success of OPAT among PWID. In a pilot randomized controlled trial for patients with OUD requiring IV antibiotics, all received treatment with buprenorphine, and those randomized to home OPAT had equal success to those receiving HBAT.[23,24] In 1 health system, an IV antibiotic risk score was implemented to assess addiction disease activity to guide OPAT decisions.[25] Using this score, low-risk patients were eligible to complete antibiotic outside the hospital, which reduced mean hospital stay by 20 days.

Applying Outpatient Parenteral Antimicrobial Therapy Data to People Who Inject Drugs

One of the key determinants in considering the implementation of OPAT for PWID is the expected efficacy of the alternatives to OPAT. In this section, the authors presume that the IDU-associated infection in question requires at least daily doses of IV antibiotics. In such cases, the alternative to OPAT is prolonged hospitalization for HBAT. Prolonged hospitalizations for PWID can be traumatic and an antitherapeutic experience.[26] These hospital stays are marked by untreated withdrawal, undertreated pain, stigmatization by health care providers, and subjection to restrictions on mobility off the ward.[27–29] Early discharge (against medical advice or AMA) is common among patients receiving HBAT, often without any antibiotics or medical follow-up, and is associated with increased mortality.[30–32] For patients who remain in the hospital, prolonged hospitalization can be a reachable moment and opportunity to initiate evidence-based therapies for SUDs.[27,33] However, addiction as the underlying cause of disease often goes unacknowledged and untreated.[30,34–37] OPAT is an effective intervention overall; success is possible among PWID, and the alternative to OPAT can be harmful and costly to patients. Effectiveness of OPAT for PWID depends on the individual patient's SUD, access to addiction treatment (including medication for opioid use disorder [MOUD], when indicated), and SNF and home infusion company acceptance of PWID receiving OPAT/MOUD.[38]

ORAL ANTIBIOTICS FOR INJECTION DRUG USE-ASSOCIATED INFECTIONS
Evidence for Oral Antibiotics for Severe Infections in the General Population

Dogma has long dictated that severe bacterial infections should be treated with IV antibiotics. The preference for IV over oral antibiotics has been especially pervasive for osteomyelitis and endocarditis, yet recent studies have shown noninferiority of oral versus IV antibiotics for common severe infections among PWID. Many of these studies focus on the use of antibiotics with high oral bioavailability or combination therapy including at least 2 agents with differing mechanisms of action. Schrenzel and colleagues[39] compared a fluoroquinolone/rifamycin combination versus fluclox-acillin or vancomycin for severe staphylococcal infections, excluding left-sided endocarditis, and showed noninferiority of the oral regimen. There are multiple retrospective studies showing noninferiority of early switch to oral antibiotics—primarily linezolid—for uncomplicated SAB and other severe S aureus infections; however, they are prone to selection bias and should be confirmed by prospective studies.[40–42]

Two recent randomized controlled trials (RCTs) for the treatment of endocarditis and osteomyelitis have led to wider adoption of oral antibiotics for severe infections. The POET (Partial Oral Treatment of Endocarditis) trial compared an early switch to oral antibiotics for patients with left-sided endocarditis caused primarily by methicillin-sensitive S aureus (MSSA), Streptococcus species, and Enterococcus species.[11] Patients with minimal valve complications were randomized to switch to oral combination therapy after at least 10 days of IV therapy or to continue on IV. The composite outcome rates were 12% in the IV arm and 9% in the oral arm, consistent with noninferiority. Long-term follow-up continued to show noninferiority of oral therapy.[43] The OVIVA (Oral Versus Intravenous Antibiotics) study was a pragmatic clinical trial comparing oral versus IV therapy for bone and joint infections performed in the United Kingdom. Patients were randomized to oral or IV therapy after less than 7 days of IV lead-in. Treatment failure at 1 year was noninferior between the 2 arms (15% IV vs 13% oral), with more catheter-related complications in the IV group.

Evidence for Oral Antibiotics for Severe Infections Among People Who Inject Drugs

Studies of oral antibiotics for severe infections among PWID date back to the late 1980s but have not been rigorously studied in the modern era. The first attempt at using oral therapy for right-sided S aureus endocarditis was documented in 1989 when a cohort of 14 patients were treated with ciprofloxacin and rifampin for 4 weeks.[44] An RCT of oral versus IV therapy for right-sided endocarditis among PWID published in 1996 showed noninferiority of oral therapy; few patients, however, had MRSA, and all remained inpatient despite receiving oral therapy.[45] Of the high-quality RCTs noted previously, few included any PWID (POET included 5 PWID) or otherwise did not report on the number of patients with SUDs (OVIVA). In an observational study of oral versus IV therapy for MRSA bacteremia, 20% (N = 99) were PWID, of which 22 received oral antibiotics.[41] Subgroup analysis of these 99 patients was not reported, but of the 5 total failures in the oral group, 2 were PWID. In sum, there is minimal contemporary data comparing outcomes of oral versus IV therapy among PWID for severe IDU-associated infections.

Applying Oral Antibiotic Data to People Who Inject Drugs

The potential benefits of oral therapy for PWID include shorter hospitalizations, more freedom, and lack of PICC-related complications. Although there is robust evidence to support the use of oral antibiotics for bone/joint infections and endocarditis, there are a few important limitations in applying these data to PWID. The use of long-term IV antibiotics often comes with weekly clinical follow-up and monitoring that might be lacking in the real-world application of oral antibiotics to PWID. In POET, patients receiving combination oral antibiotics were seen up to 3 times weekly with close follow-up of response to therapy. The health care contact that comes along with HBAT and OPAT (eg, home health nurse visits) might lead to greater adherence to IV than oral therapy. Data supporting oral antibiotics for severe infections should be applied to PWID with caution and are not a license to discharge patients with pills and minimal follow-up plans.[46] Another consideration is that oral antibiotic regimens may have more potential drug interactions relevant to PWID including the common use of rifamycins in many well-studied oral regimens (see **Table 2**). OVIVA and POET included few patients with MRSA infection, which is common among PWID in the United States.[47] Similarly, many studies used fluoroquinolone combination therapy, to which there is increasing resistance among S aureus isolates worldwide.[48] The use of oral antibiotics for severe infections among PWID is promising and can be successfully implemented, but should include shared decision making with patients, with consideration of their social situation and addiction treatment options, rather than being a 1-size-fits-all approach.

Shorter-Course Antibiotics for Injection Drug Use-Associated Infections

Increasing evidence supports the idea that traditional lengths of antibiotic therapy can be shortened substantially without compromising outcomes and with fewer antibiotic-related adverse events.[13,49,50] Most of these data have been accrued for pneumonia, urinary tract infections (UTIs), cellulitis, gram-negative bacteremia, and intra-abdominal infections, with few rigorous clinical trials evaluating short-course therapy for infections typical among PWID, such as osteomyelitis and endocarditis. A systematic review and meta-analysis of treatment length of osteomyelitis—more than half were pediatric patients—showed noninferiority of shorter course overall, with an odds ratio of 1.50 (95% confidence interval [CI] 0.97-2.34) for treatment failure; however, subgroup analyses indicated some important differences.[51] Patients with S aureus infections and those with vertebral osteomyelitis had more treatment failure when given less than 4 to 6 weeks of antibiotics. There was also no subgroup analysis of adult-only trials, which severely limits adaptation to PWID. An RCT of 2 versus 4 weeks of antibiotics for primarily small-joint septic arthritis showed noninferiority of a short course, as did a comparison of 6 versus 12 weeks for pyogenic vertebral osteomyelitis.[52,53] In contrast, a prospective observational study of treatment for hematogenous vertebral osteomyelitis showed decreasing relapse with increasing length of treatment, especially among patients with MRSA infection and undrained abscesses.[54]

Evidence for Shorter Course Antibiotics for Severe Infections Among People Who Inject Drugs

Studies of short- versus longer-course antibiotics have almost systematically not included PWID. The only 2 studies specific to PWID evaluate a shorter antibiotic course of combination therapy including an aminoglycoside for right-sided S aureus endocarditis without a longer-course comparator.[55,56] Chambers and colleagues[55] performed a prospective study and administered 2 weeks of nafcillin (N = 50) or vancomycin (N = 3) both with tobramycin to 53 PWID. They found 94% and 33% (N = 1) cure rates with nafcillin and vancomycin, respectively. Ribera and colleagues[56] performed an RCT among PWID to compare cloxacillin with versus without gentamicin for right-sided MSSA endocarditis. Cure rates were similar between the 2 groups (86%–89%, P>.2), indicating high success with short-course cloxacillin monotherapy. Of studies in the general population, only the study by Gjika and colleagues (2 vs 4 weeks for native joint septic arthritis) made mention of inclusion of PWID (N = 9 out of 154).

Applying Shorter-Course Antibiotic Data to People Who Inject Drugs

In comparison to data on oral versus IV antibiotics, the shorter- versus longer-course literature is more readily adaptable to PWID. The main caveat is that most of the data on management of osteomyelitis and septic arthritis were predicated on appropriate source control procedures. PWID with more complicated infections or multifocal infections with incomplete surgical management would call into question the applicability of shorter-course approaches. Apart from native joint septic arthritis with surgical drainage, the bone/joint literature dictates 4 to 6 weeks of antibiotics for most infections, and this seems appropriate to apply to PWID. Based on the prospective study by Park and colleagues,[54] it would be reasonable to extend treatment of hematogenous vertebral osteomyelitis to longer than 6 weeks, especially in the setting of MRSA or undrained abscesses, which might be more common scenarios among PWID. As with the oral versus IV discussion, appropriate treatment of any infection requires follow-up and monitoring for response to treatment. Whether shorter or longer courses of antibiotics are used, access to postacute care ID services is crucial and ideally could be colocalized with management of the patient's SUD.[57]

LONG-ACTING INTRAVENOUS ANTIBIOTICS FOR INJECTION DRUG USE-ASSOCIATED INFECTIONS
Evidence for Long-Acting Intravenous Antibiotics in the General Population

Dalbavancin and oritavancin are long half-life lipoglycopeptide antibiotics dosed once weekly intravenously for gram-positive infections, obviating the need for daily infusions or PICCs. Both are approved by the US Food and Drug Administration (FDA) for the treatment of SSTIs, but have been increasingly used off label for treatment of other infections. Two phase 2 RCTs have evaluated the efficacy of dalbavancin for non-SSTIs. Raad and colleagues[58] compared dalbavancin for 2 weekly doses versus 14 days of vancomycin for central line-associated blood stream infections. Dalbavancin was statistically superior to vancomycin (success rate of 87% vs 50%, P<.05), but numbers were small (N = 67); no power calculation was presented, and the vancomycin arm included 11% MSSA infections, for which vancomycin is substandard therapy. The other RCT evaluated the efficacy of 2 higher-dose weekly doses of dalbavancin for osteomyelitis, performed in Ukraine. This study showed high success rates for dalbavancin (97%) for gram-positive osteomyelitis, although methodological flaws preclude strong conclusions about efficacy versus the standard of care arm, which did not represent usual practice (vancomycin was used for MSSA, and levofloxacin IV monotherapy was used for MSSA).

Real-world applications of dalbavancin and oritavancin for non-SSTI indications describe over 200 patients treated for osteomyelitis, endocarditis, bacteremia, and prosthetic joint infections with high success rates overall, but without comparison groups and limited reporting on adverse effects.[59–64] It is unclear from these studies how many of these infections could have been treated using oral antibiotics.

Evidence for Long-Acting Intravenous Antibiotics Among People Who Inject Drugs

Since long acting lipoglycopeptides became available, there has been interest in applying these lineless antibiotics to PWID. A few retrospective cohorts have evaluated the efficacy of dalbavancin among vulnerable populations, primarily PWID. Among 32 PWID with severe *S aureus* infections treated by dalbavancin, 56% had a clinical response, 13% with clinical failure, but 31% were lost to follow up with unknown outcome.[65] Bork and colleagues[66] reported the outcome of 28 patients receiving dalbavancin for non-SSTI in Baltimore, Maryland, of whom 16 (57%) were PWID. The cohort was comprised of primarily orthopedic infections and endocarditis, with a reported cure rate of 71%, but no information on the subgroup comprised of PWID.[28] Another group in Colorado included 11 PWID with non-SSTIs, but outcomes in this subgroup were not clearly described.[67]

Applying Long-Acting Intravenous Antibiotic Data to People Who Inject Drugs

The use of long-acting (LA)-IV antibiotics among PWID have the potential to address a few important problems in the management of IDU-associated infections. Adherence to daily oral antibiotics can be difficult for PWID with ongoing drug use and unstable social circumstances. The use of LA-IV for these infections is particularly encouraging given the high osteomyelitis success rate with only 2 doses of dalbavancin.[68] Concerns regarding access to follow-up and ability to adhere to treatment plans are not significantly mitigated by the use of LA-IVs. In the cohort of PWID treated with dalbavancin for *S aureus* infections, only 53% completed the planned course of therapy.[65] Although studies have documented cost savings by allowing earlier hospital discharge with LA-IV antibiotics, the use of oral antibiotics is likely to be even more cost-effective, further weakening the rationale for LA-IV therapy.[59,67]

SURGICAL PROCEDURES FOR THE TREATMENT OF INJECTION DRUG USE-ASSOCIATED INFECTIONS
Evidence for Surgical Interventions for Severe Infections in the General Population

With the exception of 1 RCT, data for indications and timing of valve surgery for infectious endocarditis are limited to observational data and subject to survivor and selection bias.[69,70] A propensity score-matched meta-analysis of early valve surgery ($\leq$20 days) versus conventional therapy (surgery >20 days) or no surgery found early valve surgery was associated with decreased all-cause mortality compared with conventional therapy (odds ratio 0.41 [95% CI 0.31–0.54]).[69] The only randomized control trial evaluating timing of valve surgery for infectious endocarditis included patients with native left-sided infectious endocarditis who had large vegetations (>10 mm) and no urgent indication for surgery.[70] Early surgery reduced in-hospital mortality and embolic events, but not 6-month all-cause mortality. Only 8 patients in this trial had *S aureus* endocarditis, and none were reported to be PWID.

Evidence for Surgical Interventions for Severe Infections Among People Who Inject Drugs

The data on surgical outcomes for infections among PWID are primarily retrospective studies of valve surgery for IDU endocarditis. Most found that postoperative mortality among those with IDU-endocarditis and non-IDU-endocarditis was similar in the short-term.[71–73] The outcomes following the acute postoperative period among PWID appear to be worse, with 1 institution reporting a tenfold increase in mortality in the 3- to 6-month period following surgery.[72] Long-term mortality among PWID with endocarditis is high. In a cohort with a mean age of 36 years, the 10-year survival was just 44%.[7] Most deaths following valve surgery are related to ongoing IDU, and the need for reoperation was associated with increased mortality.[74] Importantly, addiction treatment referral is strongly correlated with survival among PWID with infectious endocarditis (hazard ratio 0.29).[32]

Applying Surgical Intervention Data to People Who Inject Drugs

When considering surgical interventions for PWID with severe infections, it is important to consider that even in the best circumstances, addiction is a relapsing disease, and ongoing episodes of drug use are expected.[75] In some cases, prosthetic material can be feasibly avoided, such as in tricuspid valve endocarditis. In this case, survival following tricuspid valve repair and replacement was similar, but repair was associated with lower risk for recurrent infection and need for reoperation.[76] Additionally, PWID tend to be younger, and many prosthetic devices have a finite lifespan. Thus, prosthetic material should be avoided whenever feasible, but the desire to avoid surgery should never supersede the most effective course of action to cure a severe infection. It may be true that PWID have higher medium-term mortality after endocarditis valve surgery compared with those who do not use injection drugs; however, the important unanswered question is how those with IDU-associated endocarditis would

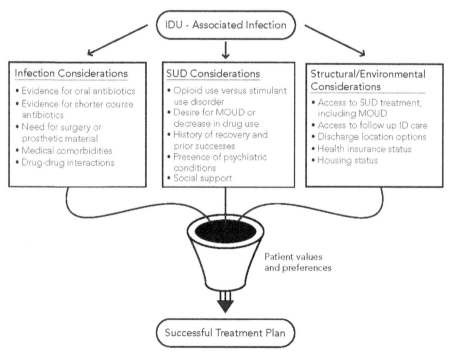

Fig. 1. Factors to consider when developing an evidence-based treatment plan for IDU-associated infections. When confronted with an IDU-associated infection, clinicians must balance the best available ID literature (infection considerations) with a patient's SUD (SUD considerations). Both must be realistic and feasible given the local environment and social circumstances of the patient (structural/environmental considerations). Finally, any successful plan must be filtered through each individual's values and preferences.

have done without any surgery. There are conflicting retrospective data on whether valve surgery is a predictor of survival in IDU-associated endocarditis.[7,32]

Application of surgical literature to PWID is also limited by the scant data on the effect of MOUD and other addiction treatments on infection-related outcomes. Most retrospective studies of IDU-associated endocarditis surgery do not report information on SUD diagnoses or utilization of MOUD. Outcomes following implementation of MOUD for patients with IDU-associated infections are being researched actively. Early reports from a cohort of IDU-associated endocarditis patients in Massachusetts indicate reduced mortality among those who took at least 3 months of MOUD following diagnosis.[77] Even without clear data on infection outcomes, MOUD should be routinely offered to patients with OUD based on strong evidence of decreasing overall mortality, retention in addiction treatment, and improved quality of life.[78]

SUMMARY

Successful management of IDU-associated infectious diseases requires a deliberate and earnest assessment of the literature and application to each unique patient. Clinical data supporting noninferiority of less-invasive, expensive, and dangerous approaches to infectious diseases should not be used as a license to deliver lower quality care to PWID. Instead, these data should be scrutinized to evaluate applicability to PWID, considering their unique challenges, before being carefully applied in practice. **Fig. 1** provides a framework for considerations and treatment decisions for patients hospitalized with IDU-associated infections. Infectious disease, SUD, and environmental domains each play a vital role in the development of an individualized successful treatment plan. Most importantly, any treatment plan must be in line with a patient's values and preferences. Future research should focus on increasing the inclusion of PWID into pragmatic clinical trials, improving assessment of SUD diagnoses and utilization of MOUD, and working on comparing interventions between PWID rather than comparing primarily with other patients.

ACKNOWLEDGMENTS

The authors would like to thank Zabrina Quidiello for graphic design assistance with the figure.

DISCLOSURE

The authors have nothing to disclose.

REFERENCES

1. Cranston K, Alpren C, John B, et al. Notes from the field: HIV diagnoses among persons who inject drugs - Northeastern Massachusetts, 2015-2018. MMWR Morb Mortal Wkly Rep 2019;68(10):253–4.
2. Zibbell JE, Iqbal K, Patel RC, et al. Increases in hepatitis C virus infection related to injection drug use among persons aged </=30 years - Kentucky, Tennessee, Virginia, and West Virginia, 2006-2012. MMWR Morb Mortal Wkly Rep 2015; 64(17):453–8.
3. Wurcel AG, Anderson JE, Chui KK, et al. Increasing infectious endocarditis admissions among young people who inject drugs. Open Forum Infect Dis 2016; 3(3):ofw157.

4. Schranz AJ, Fleischauer A, Chu VH, et al. Trends in drug use-associated infective endocarditis and heart valve surgery, 2007 to 2017: a study of statewide discharge data. Ann Intern Med 2018;170(1):31–40.

5. Ciccarone D, Unick GJ, Cohen JK, et al. Nationwide increase in hospitalizations for heroin-related soft tissue infections: associations with structural market conditions. Drug Alcohol Depend 2016;163:126–33.

6. McCarthy NL, Baggs J, See I, et al. Bacterial infections associated with substance use disorders, large cohort of United States Hospitals, 2012-2017. Clin Infect Dis 2020. https://doi.org/10.1093/cid/ciaa008.

7. Straw S, Baig MW, Gillott R, et al. Long-term outcomes are poor in intravenous drug users following infective endocarditis, even after surgery. Clin Infect Dis 2019. https://doi.org/10.1093/cid/ciz869.

8. Serota DP, Vettese T. New answers for old questions in the treatment of severe infections from injection drug use. J Hosp Med 2019;14:E1–7.

9. Rapoport AB, Fischer LS, Santibanez S, et al. Infectious diseases physicians' perspectives regarding injection drug use and related infections, United States, 2017. Open Forum Infect Dis 2018;5(7):ofy132.

10. Fanucchi L, Leedy N, Li J, et al. Perceptions and practices of physicians regarding outpatient parenteral antibiotic therapy in persons who inject drugs. J Hosp Med 2016;11(8):581–2.

11. Iversen K, Ihlemann N, Gill SU, et al. Partial oral versus intravenous antibiotic treatment of endocarditis. N Engl J Med 2019;380(5):415–24.

12. Li HK, Rombach I, Zambellas R, et al. Oral versus intravenous antibiotics for bone and joint infection. N Engl J Med 2019;380(5):425–36.

13. Spellberg B. Shorter is better. 2019. Available at: https://www.bradspellberg.com/shorter-is-better. Accessed January 4, 2020.

14. Wald-Dickler N, Holtom P, Spellberg B. Busting the myth of "static vs cidal": a systemic literature review. Clin Infect Dis 2018;66(9):1470–4.

15. Norris AH, Shrestha NK, Allison GM, et al. 2018 Infectious Diseases Society of America clinical practice guideline for the management of outpatient parenteral antimicrobial therapy. Clin Infect Dis 2019;68(1):e1–35.

16. Perica SJ, Llopis J, Gonzalez-Ramallo V, et al. Outpatient parenteral antibiotic treatment for infective endocarditis: a prospective cohort study from the GAMES Cohort. Clin Infect Dis 2019;69(10):1690–700.

17. Mitchell ED, Czoski Murray C, Meads D, et al. Clinical and cost-effectiveness, safety and acceptability of community intravenous antibiotic service models: CIVAS systematic review. BMJ Open 2017;7(4):e013560.

18. Townsend J, Keller S, Tibuakuu M, et al. Outpatient parenteral therapy for complicated *Staphylococcus aureus* infections: a snapshot of processes and outcomes in the real world. Open Forum Infect Dis 2018;5(11):ofy274.

19. Seaton RA, Barr DA. Outpatient parenteral antibiotic therapy: principles and practice. Eur J Intern Med 2013;24(7):617–23.

20. Suzuki J, Johnson J, Montgomery M, et al. Outpatient parenteral antimicrobial therapy among people who inject drugs: a review of the literature. Open Forum Infect Dis 2018;5(9):ofy194.

21. D'Couto HT, Robbins GK, Ard KL, et al. Outcomes according to discharge location for persons who inject drugs receiving outpatient parenteral antimicrobial therapy. Open Forum Infect Dis 2018;5(5):ofy056.

22. Mansour O, Arbaje AI, Townsend JL. Patient experiences with outpatient parenteral antibiotic therapy: results of a patient survey comparing skilled nursing facilities and home infusion. Open Forum Infect Dis 2019;6(12):ofz471.

23. Fanucchi LC, Walsh SL, Thornton AC, et al. Integrated outpatient treatment of opioid use disorder and injection-related infections: a description of a new care model. Prev Med 2019;128:105760.

24. Fanucchi LC, Walsh SL, Thornton AC, et al. Outpatient parenteral antimicrobial therapy plus buprenorphine for opioid use disorder and severe injection-related infections. Clin Infect Dis 2019;70(6):1226–9.

25. Eaton EF, Mathews RE, Lane PS, et al. A 9-point risk assessment for patients who inject drugs requiring intravenous antibiotics may allow health systems to focus inpatient resources on those at greatest risk of ongoing drug use. Clin Infect Dis 2018;68(6):1041–3.

26. Fanucchi LC. Do persons with opioid use disorder and injection-related infections really need prolonged hospitalizations to complete intravenous antibiotic therapy? San Francisco (CS): ID Week; 2018.

27. Velez CM, Nicolaidis C, Korthuis PT, et al. "It's been an experience, a life learning experience": a qualitative study of hospitalized patients with substance use disorders. J Gen Intern Med 2017;32(3):296–303.

28. Bearnot B, Mitton JA, Hayden M, et al. Experiences of care among individuals with opioid use disorder-associated endocarditis and their healthcare providers: results from a qualitative study. J Subst Abuse Treat 2019;102:16–22.

29. Alfandre D, Geppert C. Ethical considerations in the care of hospitalized patients with opioid-use and injection drug-use disorders. J Hosp Med 2019; 14(2):123–5.

30. Serota DP, Niehaus ED, Schechter MC, et al. Disparity in quality of infectious disease vs addiction care among patients with injection drug use-associated staphylococcus aureus bacteremia. Open Forum Infect Dis 2019;6(7):ofz289.

31. Ti L, Ti L. Leaving the hospital against medical advice among people who use illicit drugs: a systematic review. Am J Public Health 2015;105(12):e53–9.

32. Rodger L, Glockler-Lauf SD, Shojaei E, et al. Clinical characteristics and factors associated with mortality in first-episode infective endocarditis among persons who inject drugs. JAMA Netw Open 2018;1(7):e185220.

33. Trowbridge P, Weinstein ZM, Kerensky T, et al. Addiction consultation services - Linking hospitalized patients to outpatient addiction treatment. J Subst Abuse Treat 2017;79:1–5.

34. Serota DP, Kraft CS, Weimer MB. Treating the symptom but not the underlying disease in infective endocarditis: a teachable moment. JAMA Intern Med 2017;177(7):1026–7.

35. Jicha C, Saxon D, Lofwall MR, et al. Substance use disorder assessment, diagnosis, and management for patients hospitalized with severe infections due to injection drug use. J Addict Med 2019;13(1):69–74.

36. Rosenthal ES, Karchmer AW, Theisen-Toupal J, et al. Suboptimal addiction interventions for patients hospitalized with injection drug use-associated infective endocarditis. Am J Med 2016;129(5):481–5.

37. Miller AC, Polgreen PM. Many opportunities to record, diagnose, or treat injection drug-related infections are missed: a population-based cohort study of inpatient and emergency department settings. Clin Infect Dis 2019;68(7): 1166–75.

38. Wakeman SE, Rich JD. Barriers to post-acute care for patients on opioid agonist therapy; an example of systematic stigmatization of addiction. J Gen Intern Med 2017;32(1):17–9.

39. Schrenzel J, Harbarth S, Schockmel G, et al. A randomized clinical trial to compare fleroxacin-rifampicin with flucloxacillin or vancomycin for the treatment of staphylococcal infection. Clin Infect Dis 2004;39(9):1285–92.

40. Willekens R, Puig-Asensio M, Ruiz-Camps I, et al. Early oral switch to linezolid for low-risk patients with *Staphylococcus aureus* bloodstream infections: a propensity-matched cohort study. Clin Infect Dis 2018;69(3):381–7.

41. Jorgensen SCJ, Lagnf AM, Bhatia S, et al. Sequential intravenous-to-oral outpatient antibiotic therapy for MRSA bacteraemia: one step closer. J Antimicrob Chemother 2019;74(2):489–98.

42. Eliakim-Raz N, Hellerman M, Yahav D, et al. Trimethoprim/sulfamethoxazole versus vancomycin in the treatment of healthcare/ventilator-associated MRSA pneumonia: a case-control study. J Antimicrob Chemother 2017;72(9):2687.

43. Bundgaard H, Ihlemann N, Gill SU, et al. Long-term outcomes of partial oral treatment of endocarditis. N Engl J Med 2019;380(14):1373–4.

44. Dworkin RJ, Lee BL, Sande MA, et al. Treatment of right-sided *Staphylococcus aureus* endocarditis in intravenous drug users with ciprofloxacin and rifampicin. Lancet 1989;2(8671):1071–3.

45. Heldman AW, Hartert TV, Ray SC, et al. Oral antibiotic treatment of right-sided staphylococcal endocarditis in injection drug users: prospective randomized comparison with parenteral therapy. Am J Med 1996;101(1):68–76.

46. Seaton RA, Ritchie ND, Robb F, et al. From 'OPAT' to 'COpAT': implications of the OVIVA study for ambulatory management of bone and joint infection. J Antimicrob Chemother 2019;74(8):2119–21.

47. Jackson KA, Bohm MK, Brooks JT, et al. Invasive methicillin-resistant *Staphylococcus aureus* infections among persons who inject drugs - six sites, 2005-2016. MMWR Morb Mortal Wkly Rep 2018;67(22):625–8.

48. Diekema DJ, Pfaller MA, Shortridge D, et al. Twenty-year trends in antimicrobial susceptibilities among *Staphylococcus aureus* from the SENTRY antimicrobial surveillance program. Open Forum Infect Dis 2019;6(Suppl 1):S47–53.

49. Spellberg B. The new antibiotic mantra-"shorter is better". JAMA Intern Med 2016;176(9):1254–5.

50. Wald-Dickler N, Spellberg B. Short-course antibiotic therapy-replacing constantine units with "shorter is better". Clin Infect Dis 2019;69(9):1476–9.

51. Huang CY, Hsieh RW, Yen HT, et al. Short- versus long-course antibiotics in osteomyelitis: A systematic review and meta-analysis. Int J Antimicrob Agents 2019; 53(3):246–60.

52. Bernard L, Dinh A, Ghout I, et al. Antibiotic treatment for 6 weeks versus 12 weeks in patients with pyogenic vertebral osteomyelitis: an open-label, non-inferiority, randomised, controlled trial. Lancet 2015;385(9971):875–82.

53. Gjika E, Beaulieu JY, Vakalopoulos K, et al. Two weeks versus four weeks of antibiotic therapy after surgical drainage for native joint bacterial arthritis: a prospective, randomised, non-inferiority trial. Ann Rheum Dis 2019;78(8):1114–21.

54. Park KH, Cho OH, Lee JH, et al. Optimal duration of antibiotic therapy in patients with hematogenous vertebral osteomyelitis at low risk and high risk of recurrence. Clin Infect Dis 2016;62(10):1262–9.

55. Chambers HF, Miller RT, Newman MD. Right-sided Staphylococcus aureus endocarditis in intravenous drug abusers: two-week combination therapy. Ann Intern Med 1988;109(8):619–24.

56. Ribera E, Gomez-Jimenez J, Cortes E, et al. Effectiveness of cloxacillin with and without gentamicin in short-term therapy for right-sided Staphylococcus aureus

endocarditis. A randomized, controlled trial. Ann Intern Med 1996;125(12):969–74.

57. Serota DP, Barocas JA, Springer SA. Infectious complications of addiction: a call for a new subspecialty within infectious diseases. Clin Infect Dis 2019;70(5):968–72.

58. Raad I, Darouiche R, Vazquez J, et al. Efficacy and safety of weekly dalbavancin therapy for catheter-related bloodstream infection caused by gram-positive pathogens. Clin Infect Dis 2005;40(3):374–80.

59. Bouza E, Valerio M, Soriano A, et al. Dalbavancin in the treatment of different gram-positive infections: a real-life experience. Int J Antimicrob Agents 2018;51(4):571–7.

60. Tobudic S, Forstner C, Burgmann H, et al. Dalbavancin as primary and sequential treatment for gram-positive infective endocarditis: 2-year experience at the General Hospital of Vienna. Clin Infect Dis 2018;67(5):795–8.

61. Chastain DB, Davis A. Treatment of chronic osteomyelitis with multidose oritavancin: a case series and literature review. Int J Antimicrob Agents 2019;53(4):429–34.

62. Morata L, Cobo J, Fernandez-Sampedro M, et al. Safety and efficacy of prolonged use of dalbavancin in bone and joint infections. Antimicrob Agents Chemother 2019;63(5):e02280.

63. Wunsch S, Krause R, Valentin T, et al. Multicenter clinical experience of real life Dalbavancin use in gram-positive infections. Int J Infect Dis 2019;81:210–4.

64. Almangour TA, Perry GK, Terriff CM, et al. Dalbavancin for the management of gram-positive osteomyelitis: Effectiveness and potential utility. Diagn Microbiol Infect Dis 2019;93(3):213–8.

65. Bryson-Cahn C, Beieler AM, Chan JD, et al. Dalbavancin as secondary therapy for serious staphylococcus aureus infections in a vulnerable patient population. Open Forum Infect Dis 2019;6(2):ofz028.

66. Bork JT, Heil EL, Berry S, et al. Dalbavancin use in vulnerable patients receiving outpatient parenteral antibiotic therapy for invasive gram-positive infections. Infect Dis Ther 2019;8(2):171–84.

67. Morrisette T, Miller MA, Montague BT, et al. Long-acting lipoglycopeptides: "lineless antibiotics" for serious infections in persons who use drugs. Open Forum Infect Dis 2019;6(7):ofz274.

68. Rappo U, Puttagunta S, Shevchenko V, et al. Dalbavancin for the treatment of osteomyelitis in adult patients: a randomized clinical trial of efficacy and safety. Open Forum Infect Dis 2019;6(1):ofy331.

69. Anantha Narayanan M, Mahfood Haddad T, Kalil AC, et al. Early versus late surgical intervention or medical management for infective endocarditis: a systematic review and meta-analysis. Heart 2016;102(12):950–7.

70. Kang DH, Kim YJ, Kim SH, et al. Early surgery versus conventional treatment for infective endocarditis. N Engl J Med 2012;366(26):2466–73.

71. Hall R, Shaughnessy M, Boll G, et al. Drug-use and post-operative mortality following valve surgery for infective endocarditis: a systematic review and meta-analysis. Clin Infect Dis 2019;69(7):1120–9.

72. Shrestha NK, Jue J, Hussain ST, et al. Injection drug use and outcomes after surgical intervention for infective endocarditis. Ann Thorac Surg 2015;100(3):875–82.

73. Wurcel AG, Boll G, Burke D, et al. Impact of substance use disorder on midterm mortality after valve surgery for endocarditis. Ann Thorac Surg 2020;109(5):1426–32.

74. Nguemeni Tiako MJ, Mori M, Bin Mahmood SU, et al. Recidivism is the leading cause of death among intravenous drug users who underwent cardiac surgery for infective endocarditis. Semin Thorac Cardiovasc Surg 2019;31(1):40–5.

75. Schuckit MA. Treatment of opioid-use disorders. N Engl J Med 2016;375(4): 357–68.

76. Yanagawa B, Elbatarny M, Verma S, et al. Surgical management of tricuspid valve infective endocarditis: a systematic review and meta-analysis. Ann Thorac Surg 2018;106(3):708–14.

77. Kimmel SD, Walley AY, Berson D, et al. Medications for opioid use disorder following injection drug associated endocarditis. Orlando (FL): American Society of Addiction Medicine Conference; 2019.

78. Mancher M, Leshner AI. National Academies of Sciences Engineering and Medicine (U.S.). Committee on Medication-Assisted Treatment for Opioid Use Disorder. Medications for opioid use disorder save lives. In: Consensus study report of the national academies of sciences, engineering, medicine. Washington, DC: National Academies Press; 2019. Available at: https://www.ncbi.nlm.nih.gov/books/NBK538936/.

79. Leahey PA, LaSalvia MT, Rosenthal ES, et al. High morbidity and mortality among patients with sentinel admission for injection drug use-related infective endocarditis. Open Forum Infect Dis 2019;6(4):ofz089.

80. Nasa P, Juneja D, Singh O. Severe sepsis and septic shock in the elderly: an overview. World J Crit Care Med 2012;1(1):23–30.

81. Clifford KM, Dy-Boarman EA, Haase KK, et al. Challenges with diagnosing and managing sepsis in older adults. Expert Rev Anti Infect Ther 2016;14(2):231–41.

82. Antoniou T, Hollands S, Macdonald EM, et al. Trimethoprim-sulfamethoxazole and risk of sudden death among patients taking spironolactone. CMAJ 2015; 187(4):E138–43.

83. Fralick M, Macdonald EM, Gomes T, et al. Co-trimoxazole and sudden death in patients receiving inhibitors of renin-angiotensin system: population based study. BMJ 2014;349:g6196.

84. Colledge S, Larney S, Peacock A, et al. Depression, post-traumatic stress disorder, suicidality and self-harm among people who inject drugs: a systematic review and meta-analysis. Drug Alcohol Depend 2019;207:107793.

85. Mackesy-Amiti ME, Donenberg GR, Ouellet LJ. Prevalence of psychiatric disorders among young injection drug users. Drug Alcohol Depend 2012; 124(1–2):70–8.

86. Mackesy-Amiti ME, Donenberg GR, Ouellet LJ. Prescription opioid misuse and mental health among young injection drug users. Am J Drug Alcohol Abuse 2015;41(1):100–6.

87. Burnett JC, Broz D, Spiller MW, et al. HIV infection and hiv-associated behaviors among persons who inject drugs - 20 cities, United States, 2015. MMWR Morb Mortal Wkly Rep 2018;67(1):23–8.

88. Degenhardt L, Peacock A, Colledge S, et al. Global prevalence of injecting drug use and sociodemographic characteristics and prevalence of HIV, HBV, and HCV in people who inject drugs: a multistage systematic review. Lancet Glob Health 2017;5(12):e1192–207.

89. Biancarelli DL, Biello KB, Childs E, et al. Strategies used by people who inject drugs to avoid stigma in healthcare settings. Drug Alcohol Depend 2019; 198:80–6.

90. Gilbert AR, Hellman JL, Wilkes MS, et al. Self-care habits among people who inject drugs with skin and soft tissue infections: a qualitative analysis. Harm Reduct J 2019;16(1):69.

91. Monteiro J, Phillips KT, Herman DS, et al. Self-treatment of skin infections by people who inject drugs. Drug Alcohol Depend 2019;206:107695.

92. Summers PJ, Hellman JL, MacLean MR, et al. Negative experiences of pain and withdrawal create barriers to abscess care for people who inject heroin. A mixed methods analysis. Drug Alcohol Depend 2018;190:200–8.

93. Starrels JL, Barg FK, Metlay JP. Patterns and determinants of inappropriate antibiotic use in injection drug users. J Gen Intern Med 2009;24(2):263–9.

94. Linton SL, Cooper HL, Kelley ME, et al. Cross-sectional association between ZIP code-level gentrification and homelessness among a large community-based sample of people who inject drugs in 19 US cities. BMJ Open 2017;7(6): e013823.

95. Centers for Disease Control and Prevention. HIV Infection, Risk, Prevention, and Testing Behaviors among Persons Who Inject Drugs—National HIV Behavioral Surveillance: Injection Drug Use, 20 U.S. Cities, 2015. HIV Surveillance Special Report 18. Revised edition. http://www.cdc.gov/hiv/library/reports/hiv-surveillance.html. Published May 2018. Accessed January 21, 2020.

96. Meid AD, Bighelli I, Machler S, et al. Combinations of QTc-prolonging drugs: towards disentangling pharmacokinetic and pharmacodynamic effects in their potentially additive nature. Ther Adv Psychopharmacol 2017;7(12):251–64.

97. Meid AD, von Medem A, Heider D, et al. Investigating the additive interaction of QT-prolonging drugs in older people using claims data. Drug Saf 2017;40(2): 133–44.

98. Tisdale JE, Jaynes HA, Kingery JR, et al. Development and validation of a risk score to predict QT interval prolongation in hospitalized patients. Circ Cardiovasc Qual Outcomes 2013;6(4):479–87.

99. Vandael E, Vandenberk B, Vandenberghe J, et al. Development of a risk score for QTc-prolongation: the RISQ-PATH study. Int J Clin Pharm 2017;39(2):424–32.

100. Vandael E, Vandenberk B, Willems R, et al. Risk management of hospitalized psychiatric patients taking multiple qtc-prolonging drugs. J Clin Psychopharmacol 2017;37(5):540–5.

101. Gorelik E, Masarwa R, Perlman A, et al. Fluoroquinolones and cardiovascular risk: a systematic review, meta-analysis and network meta-analysis. Drug Saf 2019;42(4):529–38.

102. Bart G, Wyman Z, Wang Q, et al. Methadone and the QTc interval: paucity of clinically significant factors in a retrospective cohort. J Addict Med 2017; 11(6):489–93.

103. Ehret GB, Voide C, Gex-Fabry M, et al. Drug-induced long QT syndrome in injection drug users receiving methadone: high frequency in hospitalized patients and risk factors. Arch Intern Med 2006;166(12):1280–7.

104. Pearson EC, Woosley RL. QT prolongation and torsades de pointes among methadone users: reports to the FDA spontaneous reporting system. Pharmacoepidemiol Drug Saf 2005;14(11):747–53.

105. Baker JR, Best AM, Pade PA, et al. Effect of buprenorphine and antiretroviral agents on the QT interval in opioid-dependent patients. Ann Pharmacother 2006;40(3):392–6.

106. Katchman AN, McGroary KA, Kilborn MJ, et al. Influence of opioid agonists on cardiac human ether-a-go-go-related gene K(+) currents. J Pharmacol Exp Ther 2002;303(2):688–94.

107. Schmith VD, Curd L, Lohmer LRL, et al. Evaluation of the effects of a monthly buprenorphine depot subcutaneous injection on QT interval during treatment for opioid use disorder. Clin Pharmacol Ther 2019;106(3):576–84.
108. Litwin JS, Benedict MS, Thorn MD, et al. A thorough QT study to evaluate the effects of therapeutic and supratherapeutic doses of delafloxacin on cardiac repolarization. Antimicrob Agents Chemother 2015;59(6):3469–73.
109. Mogle BT, Steele JM, Thomas SJ, et al. Clinical review of delafloxacin: a novel anionic fluoroquinolone. J Antimicrob Chemother 2018;73(6):1439–51.
110. Lawrence KR, Adra M, Gillman PK. Serotonin toxicity associated with the use of linezolid: a review of postmarketing data. Clin Infect Dis 2006;42(11):1578–83.
111. Karkow DC, Kauer JF, Ernst EJ. Incidence of serotonin syndrome with combined use of linezolid and serotonin reuptake inhibitors compared with linezolid monotherapy. J Clin Psychopharmacol 2017;37(5):518–23.
112. Mastroianni A, Ravaglia G. Serotonin syndrome due to co-administration of linezolid and methadone. Infez Med 2017;25(3):263–6.
113. Roxane Laboratories I. Dolophine hydrochloride cii. Available at: https://www.fda.gov/media/76020/download. Accessed January 21, 2020.
114. Gillman PK. Monoamine oxidase inhibitors, opioid analgesics and serotonin toxicity. Br J Anaesth 2005;95(4):434–41.
115. Indivior. Suboxone® (buprenorphine and naloxone) sublingual film, for sublingual or buccal use CIII. 2019. Available at: https://www.suboxone.com/pdfs/prescribing-information.pdf. Accessed January 21, 2020.
116. Burdette SD, Trotman R. Tedizolid: the first once-daily oxazolidinone class antibiotic. Clin Infect Dis 2015;61(8):1315–21.
117. Kreek MJ, Garfield JW, Gutjahr CL, et al. Rifampin-induced methadone withdrawal. N Engl J Med 1976;294(20):1104–6.
118. Brown LS, Sawyer RC, Li R, et al. Lack of a pharmacologic interaction between rifabutin and methadone in HIV-infected former injecting drug users. Drug Alcohol Depend 1996;43(1–2):71–7.
119. McCance-Katz EF, Moody DE, Prathikanti S, et al. Rifampin, but not rifabutin, may produce opiate withdrawal in buprenorphine-maintained patients. Drug Alcohol Depend 2011;118(2–3):326–34.
120. Crabol Y, Catherinot E, Veziris N, et al. Rifabutin: where do we stand in 2016? J Antimicrob Chemother 2016;71(7):1759–71.

The Impact of Medications for Opioid Use Disorder on Hepatitis C Incidence Among Incarcerated Persons
A Systematic Review

Nikhil Seval, MD[a,*], Alysse Wurcel, MD, MS[b],
Craig G. Gunderson, MD[c,d], Alyssa Grimshaw, MSLIS[e],
Sandra A. Springer, MD[a,d,f]

KEYWORDS

- Hepatitis C virus • Medications for opioid use disorder • Methadone • Incarceration
- Incidence

KEY POINTS

- Hepatitis C virus (HCV) is highly prevalent in those with opioid use disorders (OUD) and in justice-involved populations.
- The data on the effect of medication treatments for OUD (MOUD eg, methadone, buprenorphine, extended-release naltrexone) on HCV incidence in prisons and jails are limited.
- MOUD effect on HCV incidence in prisons and jails was mixed in part due to the variability in each individual risk environment, suggesting the need for additional harm reduction such as syringe service programs.

Primary Funding Source: Funding for career development was received from the National Institute on Drug Abuse (K02 DA032322: Springer) and the National Center for Advancing Translational Sciences (1KL2-TR002545-01: Wurcel).

[a] Department of Internal Medicine, Section of Infectious Diseases, Yale School of Medicine, New Haven, CT, USA; [b] Department of Medicine, Division of Geographic Medicine and Infectious Diseases, Tufts University School of Medicine, 136 Harrison Avenue, Boston, MA 02111, USA; [c] Department of Internal Medicine, Section of General Internal Medicine, Yale University School of Medicine, New Haven, CT, USA; [d] Veterans Affairs Connecticut Healthcare System, 950 Campbell Avenue, West Haven, CT 06516, USA; [e] Harvey Cushing/John Hay Whitney Medical Library, Yale University, 333 Cedar Street, New Haven, CT 06510, USA; [f] Center for Interdisciplinary Research on AIDS, Yale University School of Public Health, 135 College Street, Suite 200, New Haven, CT 06510, USA
* Corresponding author. Department of Internal Medicine, Section of Infectious Disease, Yale AIDS Program, 135 College Street, Suite 323, New Haven, CT 06510.
E-mail address: Nikhil.seval@yale.edu

INTRODUCTION

There are an estimated 71 million persons globally living with hepatitis C virus (HCV) infection.[1] A significant burden of this disease is in people who inject drugs (PWID) such as opioids, and the global prevalence among PWID is estimated at approximately 40%.[2] In particular, the recent opioid epidemic has been associated with a spike in incident HCV cases among young PWID.[3] Due in part by widespread criminalization of drug use, persons who use drugs are disproportionately represented worldwide in the criminal justice system (CJS).

The confluence of incarceration, HCV, and opioid use requires evidence-based management that can address these complex and interdisciplinary public health concerns. The data on HCV transmission in the CJS, however, are limited. A systematic review evaluating HCV incidence in prisons and other closed settings meta-analyzed data from 4 sources and demonstrated a general incidence of 1.4 per 100 person-years and 16.4 per 100 person-years in detainees with a history of injection drug use (IDU).[4] Even less, however, is known about strategies to mitigate HCV transmission in this setting and their effectiveness, particularly the impact of medications for treatment of opioid use disorder (MOUD) (eg, methadone, buprenorphine, extended-release naltrexone). MOUD have been associated with a multitude of health-related outcomes including reduction in opioid use, overdose death, human immunodeficiency virus (HIV) transmission, maintenance of sustained viral response in persons with treated HCV infection, and improved HIV viral suppression in persons living with HIV.[5–11] Notably, the benefit of MOUD also includes a reduction in acquisition of HCV in the community.[12] Despite the significant evidence base, incorporation of MOUD into the global CJS has faced resistance due to stigma and cost, precluding widespread limitation. The authors undertook a systematic review with the aim of assessing the effect of MOUD on HCV incidence in prisons and jails worldwide.

METHODS

The Preferred Reporting Items for Systematic Reviews and Meta-Analyses statements for reporting systematic reviews were used for this study.[13] The study protocol was registered with PROSPERO before title and abstract review (CRD# 42019131996).

Study Selection

A systematic search of the literature was conducted in conjunction with a medical librarian in the databases Cochrane Library, Ovid Medline, Ovid Embase, PubMed, Scopus, Google Scholar, and Web of Science Core Collection to find articles published from the inception of each database until the final search on December 2019. The preliminary searches were performed in all of the databases on June 10, 2019 after being peer reviewed by a second medical librarian, and the search was repeated on December 10, 2019. The search was not limited by publication type, language, or date. Databases were searched using a combination of controlled and free text terms (**Box 1, Tables 1–5**).

Citations from all databases were imported into an Endnote X9 library. Duplicates were removed in Endnote, reducing the initial list of 3587 citations to 1939 citations. The corpus of 1929 abstracts were imported into Covidence, a screening and data extraction tool. Two independent screeners (N.S., A.W.) performed a title and abstract review with a third screener available if needed to resolve ties. The screeners selected a total of 74 records for full text review. All full articles were assessed and adjudicated for relevance by 2 independent authors (N.S., A.W.) with no resulting discrepancies.

Box 1
Search strategy

The following is the search strategy for Ovid MEDLINE to identify potentially relevant studies. MeSH headings are in bold. Additional search strategies available on request (alyssa. grimshaw@yale.edu).

1. Prisons/or prisoners/or criminals/
2. (incarcerat* or criminal justice or prison* or jail* or court* or correctional or inmate* or convict* or offender* or criminal* or penal institution* or detained or detainee or imprison* or behind bars or confinement or confined or penitentiar* or detention* or justice involve*).mp.
3. 1 or 2
4. **exp Narcotics/or exp Opioid-Related Disorders/or exp Morphine Derivatives/**
5. (opioid* or opiate* or heroin or Diacetylmorphine or diamorphine).mp.
6. OUD.ti,ab.
7. (narcotic adj3 (depend* or abuse* or addict*)).mp.
8. **Substance Abuse, Intravenous/**
9. ("injection drug use" or "intravenous drug use" or "people who inject drugs").mp.
10. (IDU or IVDU or PWID).ti,ab.
11. **exp Methadone/or exp Buprenorphine/or Naltrexone/**
12. (methadone or buprenorphine or naltrexone).mp.
13. or/4 to 12
14. 3 and 13
15. **exp Hepatitis C/**
16. (hepatitis C or hep c or PT-NANBH).mp.
17. "Parenterally-Transmitted Non-A, Non-B Hepatitis".mp.
18. (HCV or CHC).ti,ab.
19. 15 or 16 or 17 or 18
20. 14 and 19

Non-English full articles were read using Google Translate or, if needed, a colleague with native language proficiency.

Studies were included if (1) they took place in a setting of active incarceration (prison or jail); (2) there was report of MOUD received by detainees (methadone, buprenorphine, or extended-release naltrexone); and (3) there were data on either incident HCV infection or reinfection. Incidence data were to be evaluated and reported in person-year format. The authors have included studies that measured incidence by seroconversion, new viremia, or cross-sectional analysis with antibody-negative polymerase chain reaction (PCR)-positive participants as has been previously described.[14] Studies that took place in alternate settings such as community supervision (parole), detention, or noncriminal justice locations were excluded. Reviews, editorials, and commentary were also excluded. The investigators were contacted if there was any missing data such as incidence data as analyzed by MOUD receipt or for unpublished data on continually incarcerated subsets of persons. Some publications were evaluations of the same cohort over time—the most recent and inclusive sampling was identified and included in the analysis.

Table 1
PRISMA checklist

Section/Topic	#	Checklist Item	Reported on Page #
TITLE			
Title	1	Identify the report as a systematic review, meta-analysis, or both.	1
ABSTRACT			
Structured summary	2	Provide a structured summary including, as applicable: background; objectives; data sources; study eligibility criteria, participants, and interventions; study appraisal and synthesis methods; results; limitations; conclusions and implications of key findings; systematic review registration number.	2
INTRODUCTION			
Rationale	3	Describe the rationale for the review in the context of what is already known.	2
Objectives	4	Provide an explicit statement of questions being addressed with reference to participants, interventions, comparisons, outcomes, and study design (PICOS).	2
METHODS			
Protocol and registration	5	Indicate if a review protocol exists, if and where it can be accessed (eg, Web address), and, if available, provide registration information including registration number.	2
Eligibility criteria	6	Specify study characteristics (eg, PICOS, length of follow-up) and report characteristics (eg, years considered, language, publication status) used as criteria for eligibility, giving rationale.	3
Information sources	7	Describe all information sources (eg, databases with dates of coverage, contact with study authors to identify additional studies) in the search and date last searched.	2–3
Search	8	Present full electronic search strategy for at least one database, including any limits used, such that it could be repeated.	Box 1

Study selection	9	State the process for selecting studies (ie, screening, eligibility, included in systematic review, and, if applicable, included in the meta-analysis).	2–3, 15
Data collection process	10	Describe method of data extraction from reports (eg, piloted forms, independently, in duplicate) and any processes for obtaining and confirming data from investigators.	2–3, 15
Data items	11	List and define all variables for which data were sought (eg, PICOS, funding sources) and any assumptions and simplifications made.	2–3, 15
Risk of bias in individual studies	12	Describe methods used for assessing risk of bias of individual studies (including specification of whether this was done at the study or outcome level) and how this information is to be used in any data synthesis.	15
Summary measures	13	State the principal summary measures (eg, risk ratio, difference in means).	15
Synthesis of results	14	Describe the methods of handling data and combining results of studies, if done, including measures of consistency (eg, I^2) for each meta-analysis.	15
Risk of bias across studies	15	Specify any assessment of risk of bias that may affect the cumulative evidence (eg, publication bias, selective reporting within studies).	15; Table 3–5
Additional analyses	16	Describe methods of additional analyses (eg, sensitivity or subgroup analyses, meta-regression), if done, indicating which were prespecified.	15
RESULTS			
Study selection	17	Give numbers of studies screened, assessed for eligibility, and included in the review, with reasons for exclusions at each stage, ideally with a flow diagram.	Figure 1
Study characteristics	18	For each study, present characteristics for which data were extracted (eg, study size, PICOS, follow-up period) and provide the citations.	Table 6
Risk of bias within studies	19	Present data on risk of bias of each study and, if available, any outcome level assessment (see item 12).	Table 3–6
Results of individual studies	20	For all outcomes considered (benefits or harms), present, for each study: (a) simple summary data for each intervention group; (b) effect estimates and confidence intervals, ideally with a forest plot.	Table 6
Synthesis of results	21	Present results of each meta-analysis done, including confidence intervals and measures of consistency.	Figure 2

(continued on next page)

Table 1
(continued)

Section/Topic	#	Checklist Item	Reported on Page #
Risk of bias across studies	22	Present results of any assessment of risk of bias across studies (see Item 15).	Table 3–5
Additional analysis	23	Give results of additional analyses, if done (eg, sensitivity or subgroup analyses, meta-regression [see Item 16]).	20; Figure 2
DISCUSSION			
Summary of evidence	24	Summarize the main findings including the strength of evidence for each main outcome; consider their relevance to key groups (eg, health care providers, users, and policy makers).	15–19
Limitations	25	Discuss limitations at study and outcome level (eg, risk of bias) and at review-level (eg, incomplete retrieval of identified research, reporting bias).	21–24
Conclusions	26	Provide a general interpretation of the results in the context of other evidence and implications for future research.	21–24
FUNDING			
Funding	27	Describe sources of funding for the systematic review and other support (eg, supply of data); role of funders for the systematic review.	1

From Moher D, Liberati A, Tetzlaff J, Altman DG, The PRISMA Group (2009). Preferred Reporting Items for Systematic Reviews and Meta-Analyses: The PRISMA Statement. PLoS Med 6(7): e1000097. https://doi.org/10.1371/journal.pmed1000097; with permission. For more information, visit: www.prisma-statement.org.

Table 2
List of excluded articles

Year	First Author	Title	Journal	Exclusion Reason
2014	Andres	Efficacy of treatment with pegylated interferon alfa-2a plus ribavirin in prison inmates with or without personality disorder. Subanalysis of the PERSEO study	Journal of Hepatology	No reinfection data
2004	Anonymous	Canada: study provides further evidence of risk of HCV and HIV transmission in prisons	HIV/AIDS Policy & Law Review/ Canadian HIV/AIDS Legal Network	NO HCV incidence data
2009	Arora	Project ECHO (extension for community health care outcomes): knowledge networks expand access to HCV treatment with pegylated interferon and ribavirin in rural areas and prisons. Care is as effective as a university HCV clinic	Hepatology	No Reinfection Data
2001	Arrada	[Prevalence of HBV and HCV infections and incidence of HCV infection after 3, 6, and 12 mo detention in La Sante prison, Paris]	Annales de Medecine Interne	No MOUD data
2013	Asl	Outcome assessment of a triangular clinic as a harm reduction intervention in Rajaee-Shahr Prison, Iran	Harm Reduction Journal	No HCV incidence data
2010	Bate	High prevalence of late relapse and reinfection in prisoners treated for chronic HCV	Journal of Gastroenterology & Hepatology	Wrong outcomes
2013	Boelen	Molecular epidemiology and social network analysis to track HCV transmission in high-risk communities: injecting drug users in prisons of New South Wales, Australia	Journal of Hepatology	Wrong outcomes
2010	Boonwaat	Establishment of a successful assessment and treatment service for Australian prison inmates with chronic HCV	Medical Journal of Australia	No reinfection data

(continued on next page)

Table 2
(continued)

Year	First Author	Title	Journal	Exclusion Reason
2008	Brant	Diagnosis of acute HCV infection and estimated incidence in low- and high-risk English populations	Journal of Viral Hepatitis	No MOUD data
2015	Bretana	Transmission of HCV among prisoners, Australia, 2005–2012	Emerging Infectious Diseases	Duplicate study
2004	Butler	Prisoners are at risk for HCV transmission	European Journal of Epidemiology	No MOUD data
2012	Cameron	NK cell activity in exposed, uninfected prison inmates may protect against HCV	Journal of Hepatology	Wrong outcomes
2004	Champion	Incidence of HCV infection and associated risk factors among Scottish prison inmates: a cohort study	American Journal of Epidemiology	No MOUD data
2016	Chen	The excellent outcome of interferon-based HCV treatment in Taiwanese incarcerated patients	Hepatology International	No reinfection data
2008	Chong	Screening blood-borne virus among incarcerated inmates	International Journal of STD & AIDS	Wrong outcomes
2000	Christensen	Prevalence and incidence of blood-borne viral infections among Danish prisoners	European Journal of Epidemiology	No MOUD data
2017	Corless	Managing HCV infection in prison-same disease, different barriers	Gut	No reinfection data
1995	Crofts	Spread of blood-borne viruses among Australian prison entrants	BMJ	No MOUD data
1996	Crofts	Risk behaviors for blood-borne viruses in a Victorian prison	Australian and New Zealand Journal of Criminology	NO HCV incidence data
2018	Cunningham	Ongoing incident HCV infection among people with a history of injecting drug use in an Australian prison setting	Journal of the Canadian Association of Gastroenterology	Duplicate study

Year	Author	Title	Journal	Reason
2018	Cunningham	Longitudinal injecting risk behaviors among people with a history of injecting drug use in an Australian prison setting: The HITS-p study	International Journal of Drug Policy	Wrong outcomes
2017	Cunningham	Ongoing incident HCV infection among people with a history of injecting drug use in an Australian prison setting, 2005–2014: The HITS-p study	Journal of Viral Hepatitis	Duplicate study
2016	Cunningham	Stable incidence of HCV infection among people with a history of injecting drug use in an Australian prison setting, 2005–2014: The HITS-p study	Journal of Hepatology	Duplicate study
2005	Dolan	Four-year follow-up of imprisoned male heroin users and methadone treatment: mortality, reincarceration, and HCV infection	Addiction	Wrong outcomes
2010	Dolan	Incidence and risk for acute HCV infection during imprisonment in Australia	European Journal of Epidemiology	Duplicate study
2018	Farley	Ten-year durability of sustained viral response after HCV treatment in Canadian correctional institutions	Hepatology	No reinfection data
2009	Farley	The effects of treatment of HCV infection in methadone maintenance and nonmethadone maintenance	Canadian Journal of Gastroenterology. Conference: Canadian Digestive Diseases Week	No reinfection data
2011	Farley	Methadone, IDU relapse, and HCV reinfection after HCV therapy in Canadian community and inmate populations	Journal of Hepatology	No HCV incidence data
2012	Farley	Reinfection of HCV infection in HIV/HCV co-infected inmates of correctional institutions, Canada	Journal of the International AIDS Society	Duplicate study

(continued on next page)

Table 2
(continued)

Year	First Author	Title	Journal	Exclusion Reason
2011	Farley	Successful HCV treatment in correctional facilities in British Columbia, Canada: 10-y experience	Hepatology	No reinfection data
2013	Farley	Treatment response among HCV genotype 1 and their subtypes	Hepatology International	Wrong outcomes
2005	Farley	Feasibility and outcome of HCV treatment in a Canadian federal prison population	American Journal of Public Health	No reinfection data
2016	Fernandez-Gonzalez	Sofosbuvir/ledipasvir in Spanish prison population with chronic HCV	Journal of Hepatology	No reinfection data
2000	Ford	HIV, HCV, and risk behavior in a Canadian medium-security federal penitentiary. Queen's University HIV Prison Study Group	QJM	No HCV incidence data
2007	Haber	Correlates of incident HCV infection and seronegative-immune status in high risk, IDU prisoners	Hepatology	Duplicate study
1999	Haber	Transmission of HCV within Australian prisons	Medical Journal of Australia	No HCV incidence data
2017	Hajarizadeh	Incidence of HCV infection in 2 maximum-security prisons in New South Wales, Australia: The SToP-C study	Journal of Hepatology	No MOUD data
2001	Heinemann	Prevention of blood-borne virus infections among drug users in an open prison by syringe vending machines. [German]	Sucht	No MOUD data
2010	Hernandez-Fernandez	[Results of the Spanish experience: a comprehensive approach to HIV and HCV in prisons]	Revista Espanola de Sanidad Penitenciaria	No HCV incidence data
1992	Lanciani	Viral infections in a sample of intravenous drug abuser prisoners	Panminerva Medica	No HCV incidence data

Year	Author	Title	Journal	Reason
2018	Lin	Treatment of noncirrhotic incarcerated genotype 6 chronic HCV drug users, compared with genotype 1	Journal of Internal Medicine of Taiwan	No reinfection data
2008	Lloyd	Predictors of HCV incidence in IDU prison inmates	Journal of Gastroenterology and Hepatology	Duplicate study
2014	Luciani	A prospective study of HCV incidence in Australian prisoners	Addiction	Duplicate study
2004	Macalino	Prevalence and incidence of HIV, hepatitis B virus, and HCV infections among men in Rhode Island prisons	American Journal of Public Health	No MOUD data
2010	Marco Mourino	[Predictors of adherence to treatment of chronic HCV in drug-dependent inmate patients in 4 prisons in Barcelona, Spain]	Revista Espanola de Salud Publica	No reinfection data
2010	Marco Mourino	[Predictors of adherence to treatment of chronic HCV in drug-dependent inmate patients in 4 prisons in Barcelona, Spain]. [Spanish]	Revista Espanola de Salud Publica	No reinfection data
2018	Marco	Reinfection in inmates with sustained viral response after treatment of chronic HCV from 2002 through 2016 in Catalonia (Spain)	Hepatology	Duplicate study
2019	Marco	Reinfection in a large cohort of prison inmates with sustained virological response after treatment of chronic HCV in Catalonia (Spain), 2002–2016	International Journal of Drug Policy	No MOUD data
2008	Maru	Clinical outcomes of HCV treatment in a prison setting: feasibility and effectiveness for challenging treatment populations	Clinical Infectious Diseases	No reinfection data
2009	Miller	HCV infection in South Australian prisoners: seroprevalence, seroconversion, and risk factors	International Journal of Infectious Diseases	No MOUD data

(continued on next page)

Table 2
(continued)

Year	First Author	Title	Journal	Exclusion Reason
2015	Nelwan	Effect of HIV prevention and treatment program on HIV and HCV transmission and HIV mortality at an Indonesian narcotic prison	Southeast Asian Journal of Tropical Medicine & Public Health	No MOUD data
2019	Papaluca	Outcomes of treatment of HCV in prisoners using a nurse-led, statewide model of care	Journal of Hepatology	No reinfection data
2017	Papaluca	A state-wide, nurse-led model of care for HCV in the prison: high SVR12 rates that are equivalent to the specialist liver clinic	Hepatology	No HCV incidence data
2017	Papaluca	Outcomes of treatment of HCV infection in the prison setting	Journal of Gastroenterology and Hepatology (Australia)	Duplicate study
2016	Peters	HIV testing and care in prisoners: the first-year results of opt-out BBV testing in Glasgow, UK	Journal of the International AIDS Society	No HCV incidence data
2010	Pham	Frequent multiple HCV infections among injection drug users in a prison setting	Hepatology	Duplicate study
2006	Remy	Treatment of HCV in jailhouses is doable and successful: definitive data of first national French study (POPHEC)	Heroin Addiction and Related Clinical Problems	No reinfection data
2012	Rice	Comparison of HCV treatment between incarcerated and community patients	Hepatology	No reinfection data
2014	Saiz de la Hoya	Directly observed therapy for chronic HCV: a randomized clinical trial in the prison setting	Gastroenterologia y Hepatologia	No reinfection data
2010	Saksena	Treating HCV in prisoners: is it worth it?	Gut	No MOUD data
2018	Shah	Breaking free from HCV treatment in south London prisons	Hepatology	No reinfection data
2016	Simonovic	Antiviral treatment of HCV in Serbian prison setting: medical treatment outcomes and patients' adherence	Medicinski Pregled	No reinfection data

2014	Snow	Incidence and correlates of HCV infection in a large cohort of prisoners who have injected drugs	BMC Public Health	Wrong outcomes
2006	Stark	A syringe exchange program in prison as prevention strategy against HIV infection and hepatitis B and C in Berlin, Germany	Epidemiology and Infection	Wrong outcomes
2015	Szetoo	Outcome of HCV treatment in prison: a 10-y retrospective review	Journal of Gastroenterology and Hepatology (Australia)	Duplicate study
2010	Teutsch	Incidence of primary HCV infection and risk factors for transmission in an Australian prisoner cohort	BMC Public Health	Duplicate study
2015	Treloar	Acquiring HCV in prison: the social organization of injecting risk	Harm Reduction Journal	Duplicate study
2014	White	Opioid substitution therapy protects against HCV acquisition in people who inject drugs: the HITS-c study	Medical Journal of Australia	Duplicate study

Table 3
Risk of bias for cohort studies about medications for opioid use disorder effect on hepatitis C virus incidence

Author	Representativeness of Exposed Cohort	Selection of the Nonexposed Cohort	Ascertainment of Exposure	Demonstration that Outcome of Interest Was Not Present at the Start of the Study	Comparability of Cohorts on the Basis of the Design or Analysis	Assessment of Outcome	Was Follow-up Long Enough for Outcomes to Occur	Adequacy of Follow up of Cohorts	Total (/9)
Cunningham et al,[19] 2017	*	*	*	*	**	*	*	*	9
Marco et al,[20] 2014	*	*	*	*	*	*	*	-	7
Marco et al,[21] 2013	*	*	*	*	-	*	*	-	6

Average score: 7.3. Bias assessed using Newcastle-Ottawa Scale with asterisks representing stars earned for each assessment category.

Table 4
Risk of bias for randomized controlled trials about medications for opioid use disorder effect on hepatitis C virus incidence

Author	Random Sequence Generation	Allocation Concealment	Selective Reporting	Other Sources of Bias	Blinding of Participants and Personnel	Blinding of Outcome Assessment	Incomplete Outcome Data
Dolan et al,[22] 2003	Low	Low	Low	Low	Unclear	Unclear	Low

Data Extraction and Analysis

Data from the included studies were extracted by N.S. and checked for accuracy by A.W. (**Table 6**). The authors extracted crude hazard ratios from longitudinal studies that measured incident HCV infection with and without MOUD. Cross-sectional studies were not included together with longitudinal studies in the aggregated quantitative analysis.

Risk of bias was assessed for the outcome of interest in each included study using the Newcastle-Ottawa scale[15] for nonrandomized studies and the Cochrane risk of bias[16] for randomized controlled trials (RCT). The variables assessed for in comparison of cohorts were percentage of IDU, nonopioid substance use, availability of syringe service programs (SSPs), and percentage uptake of MOUD.

The effect of MOUD on HCV incidence was expressed as adjusted hazard ratios. For studies that did not report hazard ratios, the incidence rate ratio was used and calculated 95% confidence intervals. Hazard rates were pooled using random effects meta-analysis as described by DerSimonian and Laird.[17] Between-study heterogeneity was estimated using the I^2 statistic. I^2 values of 25%, 50%, and 75% were considered low, moderate, and high heterogeneity.[18] Because the number of included studies was less than 10, meta-regression or test for publication bias using a funnel plot was not performed. Statistical analysis was performed using Stata/IC, version 16.1 (StataCorp, College Station, Texas).

RESULTS

The initial and follow-up search combined returned 3857 citations in total as shown in **Fig. 1**. After removal of duplicates, 1939 citations remained. Initial title and abstract

Table 5
Risk of bias for cross-sectional studies about medications for opioid use disorder effect on hepatitis C virus incidence

Author	Representativeness of Sample	Sample Size	Non-respondents	Ascertainment of Exposure	Comparability of Different Outcome Groups	Total (/5)
Taylor et al,[23] 2013	*	*	*	*	-	4
Søholm et al,[24] 2019	*	*	*	*	-	4

Average score: 4. Bias assessed using Newcastle-Ottawa Scale with asterisks representing stars earned for each assessment category.

Table 6
Study details and outcomes

Study	Study Design	Participants	Study Size, Additional Information	Initial HCV Prevalence	Method of HCV Incidence Evaluation	MOUD Status	Total Cohort HCV Incidence	HCV Incidence with MOUD	HCV Incidence Without MOUD	Adjusted Hazard Ratio of MOUD Effect on HCV Incidence
HCV Infections										
1 Cunningham et al,[19] 2017	Prospective observational cohort	Participants from 23 correctional centers in NSW, Australia Continuously imprisoned with lifetime IDU history OR history of tattooing, piercing, blood fights. All HCV Ab negative	320 Ab-negative participants (211 in continuously imprisoned analysis) assessed from 2005 to 2014	19% on initial cohort enrolment	Biannual Ab and PCR testing	Based on "currently receiving" during biannual patient interview 15%–20% of cohort (2005–2009)	6.30/100 PY 10/100 PY among those with active IDU in prison	11.40/ 100 PY	9.60/ 100 PY	1.32 (0.43, 4.10)
2 Dolan et al,[22] 2003	Randomized controlled trial	Participants in the NSW prison system with OUD (heroin) seeking MOUD treatment	191 MMT vs 191 placebo Assessed over 4 mo from 1997 to 1998	72%–76%	HCV Ab, no PCR at 4-mo follow-up	MMT vs waitlist (4 mo)	n/a	24.30/ 100 PY	31.70/ 100 PY	0.77 (0.22, 3.56)

	Study design	Population/Setting	HCV prevalence	HCV testing	OUD treatment	HCV incidence overall	Incidence (with MMT/OST)	Incidence (without MMT/OST)	Adjusted
3 Marco et al,[20] 2014	Retrospective HCV cohort	seronegative participants in a single Barcelona prison. 2377 participants surveilled from 1992 to 2001 Annual HCV testing offered to seronegatives. Followed after release as well	"65%–99% in Spanish prisons"	HCV Ab Annual testing or with risk factors	MMT (included if continuous from enrollment to last follow-up); all persons with OUD offered MMT	1.17/100 PY[a]	1.35/100 PY (IDU with MMT)[a]	6.61/100 PY (IDU without MMT)[a]	1.07 (0.33, 3.46)
4 Taylor et al,[23] 2013	Cross-sectional study	Participants in 14 Scottish prisons. 2446 persons evaluated with Ab and PCR from 2010 to 2011 All in prison for at least 75 d	19%	HCV Ab and PCR from dried blood spot Incidence calculated based on Ab– PCR+ participants	57% of PWID on opioid agonist treatment at time of interview	0.60–0.90/100 PY overall (in-prison transmission) 3.0–4.30/100 PY among PWID	Limited 1 participant out of 479 HCV negative PWID	Limited 2 participants out of 479 HCV negative PWID	n/a
5 Soholm et al,[24] 2019	Cross-sectional Study	Participants in 8 Danish prisons. 801 persons evaluated with Ab and PCR from 2016 to 2017 All in prison for at least 75 d	9.40% serologic, 7.40% viremic	HCV Ab and PCR incidence calculated based on Ab– PCR+ participants 47% of PWID actively on MOUD	Receipt or absence of current OST asked at time of interview	0.70–1.0/100 PY overall (in-prison transmission) 18.10–24.50/100 PY among PWID	35–44/100 PY	0/100 PY	n/a

(continued on next page)

Table 6
(continued)

	Study Design	Participants	Study Size, Additional Information	Initial HCV Prevalence	Method of HCV Incidence Evaluation	MOUD Status	Total Cohort HCV Incidence	HCV Incidence with MOUD	HCV Incidence Without MOUD	Adjusted Hazard Ratio of MOUD Effect on HCV Incidence
HCV Reinfections										
6 Marco et al,[21] 2013	Retrospective cohort	Participants from 4 prisons in Catalonia, Spain. All post-HCV treatment (IFN-based) with SVR	119 participants tested annually for reinfection from 2003 to 2010 Many released in interim	n/a	Annual HCV RNA PCR Genotype assessed to confirm reinfection	All persons with IDU routinely offered low-dose MMT in prison. Linked on release and annually queried. 40% of those w/IDU on MMT throughout	5.27/100 PY[a] 33/100 PY among active IDU	1.64/100 PY[a]	7.49/100 PY[a]	0.22 (0.06, 4.14)

Abbreviations: Ab, antibody; IFN, interferon; mg, milligram; MMT, methadone maintenance therapy; NSW, New South Wales; PY, person year; SVR, sustained virologic response.
[a] Both continuously and noncontinuously incarcerated persons.

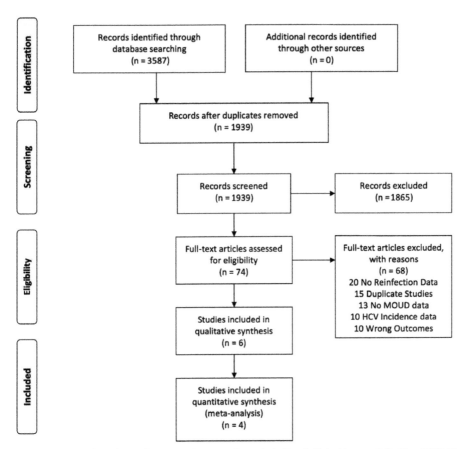

Fig. 1. PRISMA flowchart. (*From* Moher D, Liberati A, Tetzlaff J, Altman DG, The PRISMA Group (2009). Preferred Reporting Items for Systematic Reviews and Meta-Analyses: The PRISMA Statement. PLoS Med 6(6): e1000097. https://doi.org/10.1371/journal.pmed1000097. For more information, visit: www.prisma-statement.org.)

screening removed 1865 articles, and 74 articles remained for full evaluation. Sixty-eight articles were excluded, for reasons listed in **Fig. 1**. The investigators were contacted for unpublished data to determine eligibility in 16 instances. Ultimately 6 studies were included for final qualitative analysis, of which 4 were suitable for meta-analysis. Detailed study assessments and variables are reported in **Table 6**.

A total of 6 studies were included that contained data on HCV incidence reported in relation to MOUD.[19–24] Four of the studies were longitudinal analyses (3 observational, 1 RCT) and 2 were cross-sectional analyses. Two of the cohorts were based out of Australia, 2 from Spain, 1 from Denmark, and 1 from Scotland. One study described a cohort of patients who had previously been treated for HCV and retrospectively evaluated for reinfection.[21]

Hepatitis C Virus Incidence

HCV incidence in each cohort, shown in **Table 6**, varied based on geographic location and incarcerated setting. HCV incidence for subcohorts without MOUD ranged from 6.61[20] (Spain, 1990s) to 31.7 per 100 person-years[22] (Australia, 1998). HCV incidence for subcohorts with MOUD ranged from 1.35[20] (Spain, 1990s) to 24.3 per 100 person-years[22] (Australia, 1998).

All studies contained populations of incarcerated persons who were at risk of HCV acquisition and had excluded those with preexisting HCV infection. Four of the studies[19,22–24] described populations that were solely under continuous incarceration for the given analyses. The 2 Spanish cohorts[20,21] included persons who were in prison who were both continuously incarcerated and those who had been released with possible reincarceration. Investigator contact was pursued for subanalysis of HCV incidence related to MOUD in these continuously incarcerated populations but the data were unavailable.

Meta-Analysis

Of the 6 studies identified, 4 were suitable for meta-analysis[19–22] and summary incidence calculation as shown in **Table 6**. Before aggregation, HCV incidence was found to be nonsignificantly reduced in the MOUD population for 3 of the studies[20–22] and nonsignificantly increased in the MOUD population in the other.[19] When the effect of MOUD on HCV acquisition was analyzed as a hazard ratio, the pooled risk was 0.91 (0.47–1.77; $P = .505$, $I^2 = 0$) as summarized in **Fig. 2**. The cross-sectional evaluations had overall low event rates for HCV acquisition precluding accurate estimation of MOUD effect.

Substance Use and Risk Characteristics

There was a wide variability in the underlying substance use demographics of each cohort as shown in **Table 7**. Dolan and colleagues[22] had specific inclusion criteria for male prisoners with heroin use seeking methadone maintenance therapy (ie, consistent with OUD per DSM-5), and there was greater than 80% heroin use at baseline along with 40% methamphetamine use. Despite the entire cohort being actively incarcerated, continued injecting occurred during the 4-month follow-up evaluation in 75% of controls and 34% of the treatment arm. The other Australian study by Cunningham and colleagues[19] was a prospective observational cohort that enrolled in 2 discrete time periods from roughly 2005 to 2014. In the first group of enrollment, together with being HCV seronegative, all of the participants had a lifetime history

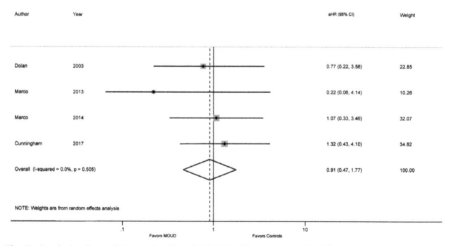

Fig. 2. Pooled adjusted hazard ratio of MOUD effect on HCV incidence.

Table 7
Study substance use characteristics

		Substance Use Characteristics	Needle/Syringe Services
1	Cunningham et al,[19] 2017	33% of total cohort reporting IDU since entering prison 18% heroin, 4% cocaine, 14% methamphetamine Also injected methadone/buprenorphine	None Bleach or quaternary amine disinfectant available
2	Dolan et al,[22] 2003	>80% heroin use at baseline 68% of treatment group still on MMT at 4-mo follow-up, 19% control subjects started MMT Average methadone dose moderate (61 mg) 40% methamphetamine use at baseline	None Bleach disinfectant available
3	Marco et al,[20] 2014	7% IDU	Yes
4	Taylor et al,[23] 2013	32% with reported lifetime history of IDU Low amount of in-prison injecting "98% of Scottish PWID inject heroin"	No
5	Søholm et al,[24] 2019	8.5% IDU 3.6% reported injecting drugs in prison No reported info on stimulant injection at time evaluation; 85% lifetime amphetamine use	No
6	Marco et al,[21] 2013	81% with life history of IDU 10.1% with active IDU during study evaluation	3 out of 4 participating prisons

Abbreviations: IFN, interferon; mg, milligram; MMT, methadone maintenance therapy.

of IDU. In the second group of enrollment, participants had either a lifetime history of IDU or another potential HCV risk factor (ie, history of tattooing, piercing, or blood fights). An overall total of 33% of individuals reported ongoing IDU since entering prison, together with 18% stimulant injection and methadone/buprenorphine injection.

The remaining 4 studies[20,21,23,24] did not specifically recruit persons with substance use but did report data on substance-using subpopulations. One Spanish cohort[20] evaluated HCV seroconversion in a single prison in Barcelona over a decade with specific subgroup analyses in persons with IDU on methadone maintenance therapy (MMT) and IDU without MMT. The overall population with IDU, though, was low, at 7%. The other Spanish cohort[21] evaluated HCV reinfection after treatment with predirect acting antiviral (DAA)-based regimens, and the lifetime IDU prevalence was 81%, although the percentage of active IDU during the study evaluation period was reported as 10.1%. Both cross-sectional studies[23,24] evaluated general inmate populations from multiple prisons and jails. In the study by Søholm and colleagues,[24] 8.5% of the population reported IDU and 3.6% reported injecting drugs in prison. The Scottish cohort by Taylor and colleagues[23] reported a 32% lifetime history of IDU, but in-prison injecting was described as "low" in frequency.

Medications for Opioid Use Disorder and Harm Reduction Characteristics

Similarly, there was wide variability in the degree of MOUD uptake in substance-using populations and availability of adjunctive harm reduction services. Cunningham and colleagues[19] reported an uptake of MMT or buprenorphine in about 15% to 20% of their originally recruited cohort with a lifetime IDU history. There were no syringe service programs in this study but bleach disinfectant materials were available. Methadone allocation was randomized in Dolan and colleagues,[22] but there was crossover reported in both study arms; 68% of the treatment group were still on MMT at 4 months, and 19% of the control subjects started MMT during the trial period. The average methadone dose was 61 mg for this study. No syringe service resources were available however. In both Spanish cohorts,[20,21] MMT was offered to all persons with IDU, and SSPs were more widely available. Marco and colleagues[21] reported in their study that 40% of those with IDU were on MMT throughout the study evaluation, and 3 out of 4 of the participating prisons had SSPs. Both cross-sectional cohorts[23,24] had moderate proportions of MOUD uptake, with Taylor and colleagues[23] reporting that 57% of PWID were on MOUD at the time of interview and Søholm and colleagues[24] reporting that 47% of the PWID were on MOUD. Neither prison system in these cohorts, however, reported using SSPs.

Hepatitis C Virus Reinfection

Only one study was identified that reported HCV reinfection related to MOUD.[21] For persons within prison with IDU reported and MOUD receipt, the HCV incidence rate was 1.64 per 100 person-years, compared with 7.49 per 100 person-years in persons within prison with a history IDU and no MOUD. Notably, although continuously incarcerated persons were included, the study was not limited to this population and included those that had been released with possible reincarceration.

DISCUSSION

The transmission of HCV virus in prisons and jails is intricately related to the carceral management of substance use disorders (SUDs) that involve IDU, in particular opioids. The authors believe their systematic review is the first to address the effect of MOUD on HCV acquisition in the justice-involved setting.

This study reveals a high degree of variability for the effect of MOUD on HCV incidence and reinfection. Despite 2 studies in the quantitative analysis suggesting a reduced HCV incidence in PWID on MOUD, the fourth study and largest cohort[19] suggested a correlation between MOUD receipt and elevated HCV incidence. As has been previously reported,[25–27] the reasons for this finding in the fourth study, known as the HITS cohort, are likely multifactorial. First, the overall MOUD uptake in their study population was relatively low. In the first half of the study, only 15% to 20% of the populations were retained on MMT or buprenorphine, all of whom had a lifetime history of IDU. Second, the HITS cohort was observational and nonrandomized, and hence those prescribed methadone or buprenorphine might represent a subpopulation of those with more severe OUD leading to more risky addiction behaviors. This was corroborated by a high degree of in-prison injecting, including approximately 18% with stimulant injection, and even injection of buprenorphine and methadone.

The range of MOUD effect on HCV incidence likely reflects the analogous range of unique risk environments that each incarcerated setting represents. In Dolan and colleagues,[22] the single RCT included in this meta-analysis, there was accordingly the least bias in MOUD allocation by virtue of randomization. HCV incidence was high, similar to the HITS cohort,[19] and a nonsignificant trend toward reduction of HCV incidence in those with methadone was reported. Both of these Australian cohorts likely represent similar risk environments with high rates of co-stimulant use and in-prison injecting. Notably, both cohorts had no SSPs. In comparison, the 2 cohorts by Marco and colleagues[20,21] had relatively lower burdens of PWID, and yet SSPs were available to the participants in most of the prisons and jails. Although this analysis was limited in power by the number of relevant included articles, further study of the MOUD effect in the presence or absence of SSPs or in terms of high versus low MOUD uptake would be informative. Whether MOUD type affects prison HCV transmission rates is also as of yet unclear. When the burden of high-risk injecting and sharing of works is substantial, implementation of factors such as high MOUD uptake and SSPs likely become more integral to reducing HCV transmission, as has been shown in nonincarcerated populations.[28] Provision of SSPs likely becomes all the more important when stimulant use is highly prevalent and MOUD is hence not effective.

For the cross-sectional studies that were not included in the quantitative analysis,[23,24] both had low overall incidences of HCV infection and limited event rates in the continuously incarcerated populations preventing assessment of MOUD effect. However, the investigators of these studies suggested that relatively low in-prison injecting populations, coupled with high uptake of MOUD (47%–57%), resulted in an overall low HCV incidence.

Relevant articles regarding the MOUD effect on HCV reinfection posttreatment in the CJS were the most limited and had the highest element of bias. In the only included reinfection study, by Marco and colleagues,[21] participants who had been treated with interferon-based regimens were surveilled with HCV RNA PCR from 2003 to 2010 on an annual basis. The overall reinfection rate was relatively low at 5.27 per 100 person-years, although this was confounded by the many persons who were released from prison during the study period. For those with IDU and on an effective dose of methadone, the incidence was 1.64 per 100 person-years compared with 7.49 per 100 person-years in those with IDU not on an effective methadone dose. Although this incidence rate difference itself was nonsignificant, the investigators found a significant difference when analyzed as a proportion (2.1% on MMT vs 16.3% not on MMT; $P = .031$). These data are similar to the extension arm of the PREVAIL study[10] that observed HCV reinfection rates as low as 1.22 per 100 person-years in a population that was fully composed of persons with OUD on agonist therapy. More data are needed to corroborate the incidence of HCV reinfection in the CJS to support feasibility of successful treatment and more widespread initiation of DAAs in prisons and jails.

Novel public health strategies are shaping the landscape of future carceral HCV management and are areas for future study on the associated impact of MOUD. Treatment as prevention and elimination of HCV from prison "microenvironments" has been successfully demonstrated, notably in one study in the context of 33% MOUD coverage for PWID and 18% of the population using SSPs.[29] HCV modeling of US prisons has shown that nationwide opt-out screening and treatment would result in a significant reduction of new infections including in the community but have been limited in their accounting for the role of MOUD and harm reduction services.[30]

Limitations

Our study was limited by the scarcity of published literature on HCV incidence in incarcerated settings, particularly in respect to its modulation by MOUD. A proportion of the full articles that were reviewed had HCV incidence data but no collection of data on OUD treatment on an individual participant level.

Efforts were made to restrict inclusion to studies that only recorded HCV incidence in continuously incarcerated persons or reported data for the continuously incarcerated population separately. Recent data have shown that the risk period after release, particularly in the acute period immediately after release, represents a different and higher risk time period in which HCV acquisition is about 60% higher than other nonjustice-involved time periods.[31] Even after contacting investigators for clarification, separate incidence data for continuously incarcerated persons were unable to be obtained for 2 of the studies included. Ultimately, though, this bias likely overestimates rather than underestimates HCV incidence reported both with and without MOUD and perhaps underestimates the MOUD treatment effect. Other mechanisms for HCV transmission, such as tattooing, anal sex, or fights with transmission of blood, would not be mitigated by MOUD therapy and could also reduce the impact of any potential treatment effect.

SUMMARY

Although this systematic review revealed a heterogenous effect of MOUD on in-prison HCV incidence, it more likely represents the varied risk environments that each incarcerated setting represents and that additional interventions such as syringe service programs are needed for incarcerated environments. Modulation of HCV acquisition is but one putative benefit of MOUD, which is a crucial evidence-based therapy that should be offered to all persons with OUD regardless of setting. The multitude of health-related outcomes, both infectious and noninfectious, are undeniable for those with opioid use disorder. There have been slow gains in the expansion of access to MOUD in incarcerated settings.[32,33] Similarly, strategies such as treatment as prevention and microelimination of HCV with direct-acting antiviral therapy are gaining recognition. Future study will be needed to best understand how to maximally care for and mitigate the risk of persons with opioid use disorder in the criminal justice system as it relates to HCV and their overall health.

CONFLICTS OF INTEREST

All authors have submitted the ICMJE Form for Disclosure of Potential Conflicts of Interest. Author S.A. Springer discloses receiving monetary compensation for scientific consultation from Alkermes Inc and receives research funding from the National Institutes of Health (NIH).

REFERENCES

1. Polaris Observatory HCV Collaborators. Global prevalence and genotype distribution of hepatitis C virus infection in 2015: a modelling study. Lancet Gastroenterol Hepatol 2017;2(3):161–76.
2. Grebely J, Larney S, Peacock A, et al. Global, regional, and country-level estimates of hepatitis C infection among people who have recently injected drugs. Addiction 2019;114(1):150–66.
3. Zibbell JE, Asher AK, Patel RC, et al. Increases in Acute Hepatitis C Virus Infection Related to a Growing Opioid Epidemic and Associated Injection Drug Use, United States, 2004 to 2014. Am J Public Health 2017;108(2):175–81.
4. Larney S, Kopinski H, Beckwith CG, et al. Incidence and prevalence of hepatitis C in prisons and other closed settings: results of a systematic review and meta-analysis. Hepatology 2013;58(4):1215–24.
5. Sordo L, Barrio G, Bravo MJ, et al. Mortality risk during and after opioid substitution treatment: systematic review and meta-analysis of cohort studies. BMJ (Clin Res Ed) 2017;357:j1550.

6. Mattick RP, Breen C, Kimber J, et al. Buprenorphine maintenance versus placebo or methadone maintenance for opioid dependence. Cochrane Database Syst Rev 2014;(2):CD002207.

7. Springer SA, Di Paola A, Azar MM, et al. Extended-Release Naltrexone Improves Viral Suppression Among Incarcerated Persons Living With HIV With Opioid Use Disorders Transitioning to the Community: Results of a Double-Blind, Placebo-Controlled Randomized Trial. J Acquir Immune Defic Syndr (1999) 2018;78(1): 43–53.

8. Springer SA, Di Paola A, Barbour R, et al. Extended-release Naltrexone Improves Viral Suppression Among Incarcerated Persons Living with HIV and Alcohol use Disorders Transitioning to the Community: Results From a Double-Blind, Placebo-Controlled Trial. J Acquir Immune Defic Syndr (1999) 2018;79(1):92–100.

9. Springer SA, Qiu J, Saber-Tehrani AS, et al. Retention on buprenorphine is associated with high levels of maximal viral suppression among HIV-infected opioid dependent released prisoners. PLoS One 2012;7(5):e38335.

10. Akiyama MJ, Lipsey D, Heo M, et al. Low Hepatitis C Reinfection Following Direct-Acting Antiviral Therapy Among People Who Inject Drugs on Opioid Agonist Therapy. Clin Infect Dis 2019;70(12):2695–702.

11. Rosenthal ES, Silk R, Mathur P, et al. Concurrent Initiation of Hepatitis C and Opioid Use Disorder Treatment in People Who Inject Drugs. Clin Infect Dis 2020;ciaa105.

12. Platt L, Minozzi S, Reed J, et al. Needle and syringe programmes and opioid substitution therapy for preventing HCV transmission among people who inject drugs: findings from a Cochrane Review and meta-analysis. Addiction 2018; 113(3):545–63.

13. Liberati A, Altman DG, Tetzlaff J, et al. The PRISMA statement for reporting systematic reviews and meta-analyses of studies that evaluate health care interventions: explanation and elaboration. Ann Intern Med 2009;151(4):W65–94.

14. Page-Shafer K, Pappalardo BL, Tobler LH, et al. Testing strategy to identify cases of acute hepatitis C virus (HCV) infection and to project HCV incidence rates. J Clin Microbiol 2008;46(2):499–506.

15. Wells G, Shea B, O'Connell D, et al. The Newcastle-Ottawa Scale (NOS) for assessing the quality of nonrandomised studies in meta-analyses. Available at: http://www.ohri.ca/programs/clinical_epidemiology/oxford.asp. Accessed December 12, 2019.

16. Higgins JP, Altman DG, Gotzsche PC, et al. The Cochrane Collaboration's tool for assessing risk of bias in randomised trials. BMJ (Clin Res Ed) 2011;343:d5928.

17. DerSimonian R, Laird N. Meta-analysis in clinical trials. Control Clin Trials 1986; 7(3):177–88.

18. Higgins JP, Thompson SG, Deeks JJ, et al. Measuring inconsistency in meta-analyses. BMJ (Clin Res Ed) 2003;327(7414):557–60.

19. Cunningham EB, Hajarizadeh B, Bretana NA, et al. Ongoing incident hepatitis C virus infection among people with a history of injecting drug use in an Australian prison setting, 2005-2014: The HITS-p study. J Viral Hepat 2017;24(9):733–41.

20. Marco A, Gallego C, Cayla JA. Incidence of hepatitis C infection among prisoners by routine laboratory values during a 20-year period. PLoS One 2014;9(2): e90560.

21. Marco A, Esteban JI, Sole C, et al. Hepatitis C virus reinfection among prisoners with sustained virological response after treatment for chronic hepatitis C. J Hepatol 2013;59(1):45–51.

22. Dolan KA, Shearer J, MacDonald M, et al. A randomised controlled trial of methadone maintenance treatment versus wait list control in an Australian prison system. Drug Alcohol Depend 2003;72(1):59–65.

23. Taylor A, Munro A, Allen E, et al. Low incidence of hepatitis C virus among prisoners in Scotland. Addiction 2013;108(7):1296–304.

24. Søholm J, Holm DK, Mossner B, et al. Incidence, prevalence and risk factors for hepatitis C in Danish prisons. PLoS One 2019;14(7):e0220297.

25. Teutsch S, Luciani F, Scheuer N, et al. Incidence of primary hepatitis C infection and risk factors for transmission in an Australian prisoner cohort. BMC Public Health 2010;10:633.

26. Dolan K, Teutsch S, Scheuer N, et al. Incidence and risk for acute hepatitis C infection during imprisonment in Australia. Eur J Epidemiol 2010;25(2):143–8.

27. Luciani F, Bretana NA, Teutsch S, et al. A prospective study of hepatitis C incidence in Australian prisoners. Addiction 2014;109(10):1695–706.

28. Palmateer NE, Taylor A, Goldberg DJ, et al. Rapid decline in HCV incidence among people who inject drugs associated with national scale-up in coverage of a combination of harm reduction interventions. PLoS One 2014;9(8):e104515.

29. Cuadrado A, Llerena S, Cobo C, et al. Microenvironment eradication of hepatitis C: a novel treatment paradigm. Am J Gastroenterol 2018;113(11):1639–48.

30. He T, Li K, Roberts MS, et al. Prevention of hepatitis C by screening and treatment in U.S. prisons. Ann Intern Med 2016;164(2):84–92.

31. Stone J, Fraser H, Lim AG, et al. Incarceration history and risk of HIV and hepatitis C virus acquisition among people who inject drugs: a systematic review and meta-analysis. Lancet Infect Dis 2018;18(12):1397–409.

32. Nunn A, Zaller N, Dickman S, et al. Methadone and buprenorphine prescribing and referral practices in US prison systems: results from a nationwide survey. Drug Alcohol Depend 2009;105(1–2):83–8.

33. Pesce vs. Coppinger, 355 F. Supp. 3d 35 (D. Mass. 2018).

Treating Opioid Use Disorder and Related Infectious Diseases in the Criminal Justice System

Daniel Winetsky, MD, MS[a,b,*], Aaron Fox, MD[c],
Ank Nijhawan, MD, MPH, MSCS[d], Josiah D. Rich, MD, MPH[e,f]

KEYWORDS

- Opioid use disorder • HIV infection • Hepatitis C virus infection
- Criminal justice involvement • Harm reduction • Methadone • Buprenorphine
- Extended-release naltrexone

KEY POINTS

- Opioid use disorder and its infectious complications are highly prevalent among criminal justice populations.
- Incarcerated patients with opioid use disorder, human immunodeficiency virus, and hepatitis C virus should be provided with medical treatment in line with the community standard of care.
- For opioid use disorder and chronic infections, screening practices and access to medications vary widely among correctional facilities.
- The transition from a correctional setting to the community represents a highly vulnerable period, marked by high rates of relapse to substance use, loss to medical follow up for human immunodeficiency virus and other infections, and fatal overdose.
- A patient-centered approach can promote health and improve engagement with medical treatment for opioid use disorder and its infectious complications.

[a] Division of Infectious Diseases, Department of Internal Medicine, Columbia University Irving Medical Center, 622 West 168th Street, PH 8 W-876, New York, NY 10032, USA; [b] HIV Center for Clinical and Behavioral Studies at Columbia University and New York State Psychiatric Institute, New York, NY, USA; [c] Department of Internal Medicine, Montefiore Medical Center, 305 East 161th Street, Room 4, Bronx, NY, USA; [d] Division of Infectious Diseases, Department of Internal Medicine, University of Texas Southwestern Medical Center, 5323 Harry Hines Boulevard, Dallas, TX 75390, USA; [e] Department of Medicine, Brown University, 164 Summit Avenue, Providence, RI 02906, USA; [f] Department of Epidemiology, Brown University, 164 Summit Avenue, Providence, RI 02906, USA
* Corresponding author.
E-mail address: dw2787@cumc.columbia.edu

Infect Dis Clin N Am 34 (2020) 585–603
https://doi.org/10.1016/j.idc.2020.06.012
0891-5520/20/© 2020 Elsevier Inc. All rights reserved.

id.theclinics.com

From 2010 to 2019, the prevalence of opioid use and incidence of opioid-related overdose increased sharply in the United States.[1,2] Fatal drug overdoses now exceed the peak mortality related to AIDS in 1995,[3] with more than 70,000 overdose deaths in 2017, approximately 47,600 of which were attributed to opioids.[4] Infectious complications of injection drug use have also risen during this time, including severe bacterial infections and chronic hepatitis C virus (HCV).[5,6] The increase in the misuse of prescription opioids[7] and the role of illicit fentanyl and its analogues[8] have often taken center stage in media coverage about the shifts in opioid epidemiology. However, a closer examination reveals a more complex picture, with multiple overlapping social and economic factors contributing to the increasing prevalence of opioid use and worsening vulnerability of people who use them.[1,9] In particular, opioid misuse and use disorder are strongly associated with criminal justice involvement.[9] Furthermore, the shifting demographics and epidemiology of opioid use have coincided with a public reexamination of systemic racism and mass incarceration, bringing renewed attention to the public health impact of criminal justice involvement. Recent estimates suggest that 1.9 million Americans have an opioid use disorder (OUD),[10] and 6.6 million are under the supervision of adult correctional systems.[11] Because both criminal justice involvement and OUD are highly prevalent and associated with comorbid infections, the delivery of care for addiction and its infectious complications within criminal justice-based health systems has wide-reaching implications, including for community-based providers of care for infectious diseases.

CRIMINAL JUSTICE INSTITUTIONS AND PUBLIC HEALTH

The "criminal justice system" is a network of separate yet interrelated public institutions, including law enforcement agencies; courts; correctional institutions, which incarcerate individuals as part of pretrial detention or sentencing for a criminal conviction; and community supervision agencies, which administer restrictions and enforce sanctions for criminal defendants who remain in the community (eg, probation, parole, and alternative sentencing programs). Among settings of incarceration, the term "jail" refers to institutions designed to hold criminal defendants in pretrial detention, while awaiting adjudication of their charges. Jails are generally administered by a local county government or sheriff's department. Prisons are usually state or federal institutions that hold individuals who have been sentenced for a criminal conviction. In some jurisdictions, shorter sentences (typically of less than 1–2 years) may be served in local jails instead of prison.[12]

The distinction between correctional institutions necessitates different models of health care delivery. For example, clinicians in county jails typically care for a highly transient patient population, often with acute medical issues occurring around the time of arrest (eg, withdrawal from substances, mental health crises, etc). Although medical service providers in jails have an opportunity to screen patients for chronic diseases (**Table 1**), establishing a plan for referral to appropriate care in the community will be a central priority for the majority of individuals. In contrast, medical care in prison will commonly include population-wide chronic disease management, health screenings, and preventive care. Regardless of the setting, however, populations with criminal justice involvement are disproportionately affected by chronic health conditions, including hypertension,[13] cardiovascular disease,[13] diabetes mellitus,[13] severe mental illness,[14] post-traumatic stress disorder,[15] OUD and other substance use disorders (SUDs),[14] human immunodeficiency virus (HIV)/AIDS,[13] and viral hepatitis.[13] Nationwide, an estimated 64.5% of those in settings of incarceration have a SUD, and 32.9% have been diagnosed with a mental health disorder.[14]

Table 1
Recommendations for preventive care among people who use opioids in the criminal justice system

Screening		Vaccination		Harm Reduction	
Disease	Recommendations	Disease	Recommendations	Disease	Recommendations
HIV	Opt-out screening on intake for all individuals[55]	Tetanus	Td recommended every 10 y and TDaP once for all adults (especially important for people who inject drugs given ongoing risk)[77]	Blood-borne pathogens	Avoid sharing of needles and equipment (including cottons, cookers, etc) Avoid using syringes to avoid drugs Smoke, snort, swallow, or "booty bump" (rectal administration) drugs instead of injecting Reduce number of sharing partners
HBV	HBsAg, HBsAb, and HBcAb recommended for all people who inject drugs[77]	HBV	Administer vaccine series to all people who inject drugs without evidence of HBV immunity (negative HBsAg)[77]	Severe bacterial infections	Use a new needle every time (avoid even personal reuse) Wash hands, use gloves and sterilize injection sites with alcohol before every use Avoid licking needles or other equipment before injection
HCV	Opt-out screening on intake for all individuals (authors' opinion and USPSTF recommendation to screen all adults)[76]	HAV	Administer vaccine with booster dose at 6 mo to all people who inject drugs (serology not necessary before vaccination)[77]	Overdose	Naloxone distribution Use a small test dose to assess drug potency before use Avoid using alone Avoid mixing opioids with benzodiazepines or other sedating drugs Counseling regarding overdose risk associated with loss of tolerance and cue-associated cravings upon release from incarceration
STDs	Screen all people who use drugs for chlamydia, gonorrhea, and syphilis[77]	Other: HPV, Pneumococcus, Meningococcus, Pertussis	As indicated based on age and HIV status		
Latent TB infection	Annual PPD or interferon-gamma release assay[84]	Seasonal influenza	Indicated annually for all adults		

Abbreviations: HBsAb, hepatitis B surface antibody; HBsAg, hepatitis B surface antigen; HPV, human papillomavirus; STD, sexually transmitted disease; TB, tuberculosis.

Because jails and prisons place individuals in confinement, they have a legal obligation to provide medical care to those under their custody.[16] A seminal 1976 US Supreme Court case *Estelle v Gamble* established that denying medical care was "deliberate indifference" to the health of incarcerated individuals and prohibited by the constitution.[16] However, people under community supervision also carry a high burden of OUD and chronic infectious diseases, but have less frequently been targeted for medical interventions. Those under community supervision typically continue to receive medical care in the community, although in some cases an individual may be mandated to participate in a particular treatment program for substance use or mental health.[12]

The relationship between criminal justice involvement and chronic health conditions is complex and multidirectional. Because of drug prohibition and the occurrence of "acquisitive crime" to sustain substance use, people with SUDs experience ongoing risk of criminal justice involvement. Furthermore, substance use and HIV have been described as being "syndemic" with interpersonal violence among economically disadvantaged communities, thereby increasing risk of criminal justice involvement.[17] Before arrest, people with criminal justice involvement are thus more likely to have experienced violence, substance use and their infectious and psychiatric sequelae and often face significant barriers to health care access in the community. Incarceration also leads to loss of housing and employment and severs social ties, thereby destabilizing people with SUDs. Overall mortality is 8 to 12 times greater than that of the general population in the early postrelease period.[18] Among people who inject drugs, sharing of needles and equipment and the incidence of HIV and HCV increase after release from incarceration.[19,20] Furthermore, a history of recent incarceration seems to be associated with increased intensity of opioid and other substance use.[9]

THE UNIQUE CHALLENGES OF PROVIDING CARE IN CORRECTIONAL SETTINGS

Health care providers working in correctional settings face unique challenges. The movement of patients and staff between physical locations is constrained and resource limitations are common within correctional health systems. Maintaining confidentiality can be challenging, because security staff are necessarily involved in patient flows and remain in close proximity to potentially violent patients.[21] The cost and discomfort associated with transporting patients to providers outside of a facility (typically in shackles and accompanied by at least 2 armed guards) also can present a barrier to receiving appropriate specialty care.[22] In particular, for people using opioids, the risk of legal sanctions for possession or unsupervised opioid use may serve as a barrier to seeking OUD treatment during incarceration.

In these and other ways, priorities set by security staff can have a powerful impact on health care delivery. At times, such as when a physical altercation occurs, the security mission of the institution must take precedence over routine medical care to protect the safety of both staff and patients. However, the security mission can also challenge professional ethics through dual loyalty, meaning that health care staff must subjugate patient care needs to security staff mandates. For example, health care staff are commonly asked to medically "clear" individuals before they are transferred to administrative segregation (ie, "solitary confinement"), which is associated with mental health risks. Addressing dual loyalty systematically with training to recognize and manage ethical conflicts, has been demonstrated to be feasible and acceptable.[23]

Prescribing decisions in correctional facilities, especially regarding medications for OUD (MOUD), are influenced by dual loyalty, security mandates, and stigma. Medical care in correctional settings is often structured to minimize the diversion of psychoactive substances such as opioid analgesics and MOUD (eg, methadone and buprenorphine), even in the face of great medical need. Although data are limited, available reports describe a predominance of psychosocial treatments and peer recovery supports (eg, alcoholics anonymous), although few correctional facilities offer MOUD.[24] Even, when MOUD is available, medications are often provided exclusively for the management of acute withdrawal, chronic pain, or for the maintenance treatment of OUD in pregnant women.[24] A preference by criminal justice staff for psychosocial drug treatment is commonly cited as a barrier to offering MOUD.[24,25] However, these attitudes contradict the community standard of care, in which psychosocial treatments combined with maintenance pharmacotherapy using methadone, buprenorphine, or naltrexone is considered first line.[26]

PATIENT-CENTERED OPIOID USE DISORDER CARE FOR CRIMINAL JUSTICE-INVOLVED PATIENTS

The ideal approach to managing OUD during incarceration requires screening, withdrawal management, initiation, or continuation of MOUD, and planning for reentry (**Figs. 1** and **2**). Most jails and prisons in the United States do not offer MOUD, but law suits, new legislation, and changes in attitudes toward MOUD are contributing to increased MOUD availability.[27] Identifying people with OUD can be challenging during incarceration, owing to the fear of further criminal sanctions for ongoing use. The Rapid Opioid Dependence Screen was recently developed and validated for use in criminal justice settings and may be a helpful tool for integrating OUD engagement into routine medical care.[28] Other validated screening instruments also exist. An initial assessment of people found to have OUD should include (1) an assessment of comorbid medical and psychiatric conditions, (2) a careful evaluation for withdrawal from opioids and other substances, (3) counseling regarding expectations for OUD management (either withdrawal management or maintenance treatment), and (4) screening for infectious and other complications of addiction. Offering the full array of MOUD options to people with OUD in criminal justice settings is feasible, safe, and effective.[29–31] Initiating and maintaining MOUD treatment during incarceration increases retention in treatment in the community after release, which results in long-term benefits, including decreased injection behavior, heroin use, and nonfatal overdose 12 months after release.[30]

Maintenance Treatment

A comprehensive OUD treatment program will provide access to full agonist (methadone), partial agonist (buprenorphine), and antagonist (extended-release naltrexone) pharmacotherapies in combination with psychosocial treatment (see **Fig. 2**). In accordance with the community standard of care, the choice of medication involves shared decision making, taking into account the patient's preferences, treatment goals, and the risks and benefits of each option.[26] In the first 18 months of a newly established program in the Rhode Island Department of Corrections, there was a 350% increase in MOUD uptake, with more than one-half of patients choosing methadone, a substantive minority (approximately 40%–45%) choosing buprenorphine and 2.5% or fewer choosing naltrexone.[29,32] Rollout of this program was associated with a decrease in opioid overdose deaths among community-dwelling individuals with recent criminal justice involvement across the state of Rhode Island.[33] These findings are consistent with international data demonstrating that receiving MOUD during incarceration is associated with large reductions in overall and overdose-related mortality during

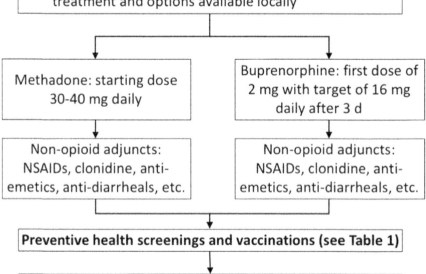

incarceration and after release.[31] In their review of this and other data, the National Academies of Science, Engineering and Medicine concluded that all medications approved by the US Food and Drug Administration for the maintenance treatment of OUD should be made available in criminal justice settings.[34]

Medical Management of Opioid Withdrawal

Under current circumstances, limited MOUD availability creates obstacles for providing the community standard of care to patients with OUD in criminal justice settings. When maintenance opioid agonist therapy is unavailable, patients with OUD will almost universally experience withdrawal upon being taken into custody. Medically managed withdrawal (often referred to as "detoxification") should be provided in these settings to avoid untreated symptoms, but clinicians must be aware this does not constitute long-term OUD treatment and is associated with an increased risk of subsequent overdose related to loss of tolerance.[35] Comparable with the management of withdrawal syndromes upon hospital admission, several options are available for symptomatic treatment (see **Fig. 1**).[36] Where possible, withdrawal management with methadone or buprenorphine is preferable (sample protocols for buprenorphine induction are available at https://pcssnow.org/wp-content/uploads/2014/02/PCSS-MATGuidanceBuprenorphineInduction.Casadonte.pdf and https://www.asam.org/docs/default-source/education-docs/clinic-induction-protocol-example_it-matttrs_8-28-2017.pdf?sfvrsn=a30640c2_2). In general, slowly tapering opioids is preferable—longer periods of time for tapering will lessen opioid withdrawal symptoms. Nonopioid adjuncts for symptom control can be used in addition to opioids (or alone if opioids are not available for withdrawal management). These include clonidine, nonsteroidal anti-inflammatory drugs, antiemetics, antidiarrheal agents, and the judicious use of benzodiazepines.[36] Careful assessment for concurrent withdrawal from other substances is critical, because benzodiazepine and alcohol withdrawal can be fatal.

The chosen approach to OUD and withdrawal management in correctional settings can have lasting effects on patient engagement in the community. In particular, the prolonged withdrawal syndrome experienced by those who are forced to taper off methadone maintenance therapy during incarceration can result in a later aversion to methadone as a treatment modality.[37] Conversely, emphasizing detoxification and avoidance of maintenance opioids can contribute to a perception of a period of abstinence in prison as a "clean time."[38] Although patients may prefer to avoid opioids and MOUD during periods of incarceration, the perspective that prolonged abstinence in correctional facilities can increase one's chances of sustaining a long-term recovery in the community is at odds with data showing that approximately 65% to 90% of people with OUD will relapse within 6 months of release in the absence of maintenance MOUD treatment, with at most a marginal benefit from prolonged abstinence.[39,40] Furthermore, a focus on the purported benefits of prolonged abstinence during incarceration may provide unrealistic expectations about the severity of cue-associated

---

Fig. 1. Approach to the patient with OUD upon intake to a correctional facility. Upon intake to a correctional facility, patients suspected of having OUD should undergo a comprehensive evaluation, including medical management of withdrawal symptoms; infectious disease screening; counseling and education; and the formulation of a plan for transition to ongoing care for OUD and its infectious complications. NSAIDs, nonsteroidal anti-inflammatory drugs; RODS, rapid opioid dependence screen.[28]

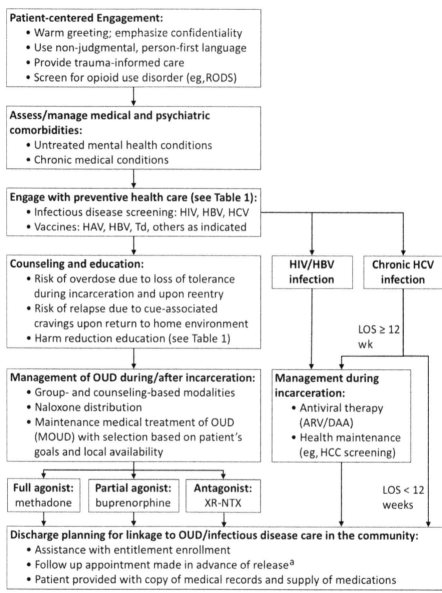

Fig. 2. Approach to the patient with OUD during incarceration and before community reentry. During incarceration, patients with OUD should undergo a comprehensive evaluation. This evaluation should include: the assessment and management of psychiatric/medical comorbidities; infectious diseases screening and immunizations; medical treatment of OUD and chronic infections; and a plan for transition to ongoing care for OUD and its infectious complications in the community upon reentry. ARV, antiretroviral therapy for HIV; DAA, direct-acting antiviral therapy for viral hepatitis; HBV, hepatitis B virus; HCV, hepatitis C virus; HIV, human immunodeficiency virus; LOS, Length of stay; RODS, Rapid Opioid Dependence Screen[28]; XR-NTX; extended-release naltrexone. [a] Patient navigation or follow-up in a transitions clinic, if available, may improve health care engagement.[61,64] (*Adapted from* Masyukova MI., Hanna DB., Fox AD. HIV treatment outcomes among formerly

cravings when patients with OUD return to their home environment. Forced withdrawal during incarceration also removes the protective effect of opioid tolerance and leaves individuals susceptible to overdose upon release if they return to using the amount that they were previously using.[35] Return to opioid use can also occur during incarceration; hence, it is critical that correctional health care systems create conditions for overdose preparedness. Necessary actions include ensuring naloxone availability in code kits, training nursing staff to administer naloxone, and establishing nurse-driven protocols for its use during an emergency in the absence of an ordering provider. Security staff may even carry naloxone and be trained in its use.[41] Correctional facilities can also distribute naloxone and provide training for its use to people reentering the community.[42]

Care During Reentry

In the early postrelease period, the risk of fatal overdose is more than 10 times that of the general population, and is greatest (>120 times the general population rate) during the first week (**Fig. 3**).[18] Therefore, any medical encounter with a patient who uses opioids during the course of incarceration presents an opportunity to provide education about the postrelease risk of overdose. Counseling can also suggest methods to reduce the risk of acquired infection in the event of relapse (see **Table 1**). Extended-release naltrexone, a long-acting, monthly injection of an opioid antagonist, decreases relapse and nonfatal overdose in people with OUD and criminal justice involvement.[40] It is particularly appealing to criminal justice institutions, because it has been marketed as supporting an abstinence-based recovery.[43] However, emerging data suggest that extended-release naltrexone may be less effective than opioid agonist therapy at protecting patients from overdose,[44,45] and its relatively limited use outside of correctional institutions may be a barrier to continuing treatment after release. The initiation of opioid agonist therapy upon release or during parole[46] is also feasible and has been shown to improve rates of viral suppression among HIV-positive people with OUD.[47] Initiating MOUD treatment at least 30 days before release has been recommended by the American Society for Addiction Medicine.[26]

INTEGRATING CARE FOR ADDICTION AND INFECTIOUS DISEASES AMONG CRIMINAL JUSTICE-INVOLVED POPULATIONS

Although OUD treatment is challenging in correctional settings, incarceration nevertheless provides an opportunity to screen, prevent, and treat the chronic infectious complications of OUD. Conversely, owing to limited access to safe injection equipment, poorly controlled OUD may lead to acute infections during incarceration. Clinicians in criminal justice settings must therefore be vigilant for infections related to substance use.

The integration of OUD treatment into infectious disease specialty care is occurring in community settings and should be the ideal during incarceration.[48] These efforts largely center around maximizing opportunities to offer MOUD during episodes of

incarcerated transitions clinic patients in a high prevalence setting. Health Justice 2018;6(1):16. https://doi.org/10.1186/s40352-018-0074-5; Cunningham WE., Weiss RE., Nakazono T., et al. Effectiveness of a Peer Navigation Intervention to Sustain Viral Suppression Among HIV-Positive Men and Transgender Women Released From Jail: The LINK LA Randomized Clinical Trial. JAMA Internal Medicine 2018;178(4):542; with permission.)

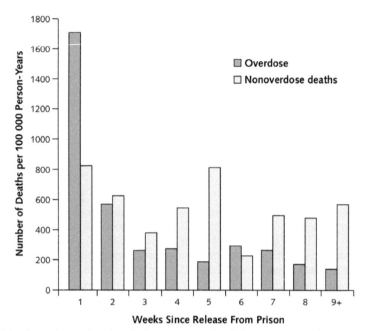

Fig. 3. Risk of overdose-related and all-cause mortality following release from prison. (*From* Binswanger IA., Blatchford PJ., Mueller SR., et al. Mortality After Prison Release: Opioid Overdose and Other Causes of Death, Risk Factors, and Time Trends From 1999 to 2009. Annals of Internal Medicine 2013;159(9):592; with permission.)

care for infections such as endocarditis, osteomyelitis, bacteremia, HIV, and HCV.[48] In correctional health care, however, specialists often have a somewhat circumscribed role. Patients cannot self-refer to specialty care, and specialist referral is often subject to strict controls to decrease the cost of care. Furthermore, the constrained movement of clinicians in correctional settings has facilitated the innovative use of telemedicine to manage chronic infections such as HIV and HCV (eg, project ECHO).[49,50] Although telemedicine allows infectious disease specialists to provide expert care for patients who are geographically dispersed across multiple facilities, it also limits their role to consultation; each facility's on-site provider is typically responsible for enacting recommendations and monitoring a patient's response between scheduled telemedicine sessions. Hence, correctional health systems must identify opportunities to integrate screening, management and preventive care protocols for both OUD and infectious diseases at the primary care level.

Acute Infections

Infectious disease specialists practicing in the community may care for incarcerated patients who become hospitalized. It is important for these providers to note that, for many people with OUD and other SUDs, illicit drug use may continue during incarceration.[51] Therefore, it is critical to take a careful substance use history, including recent injection for any patient presenting from correctional facilities with skin and soft tissue infections, osteomyelitis, endocarditis, and other endovascular infections. In most correctional institutions, medical facilities will include an infirmary, in which round-the-clock nursing care can be provided. Typically, patients will be placed in an infirmary upon return from hospitalization or admitted directly to the infirmary for observation and management of acute medical issues requiring an intermediate level of care. In many facilities, patients needing ongoing intravenous antibiotics or wound care after hospitalization remain in the infirmary for the duration of their course, mirroring the function of an outpatient parenteral antimicrobial therapy service.[52] It is essential to communicate the recommendations for clinical monitoring and further management clearly, ideally through direct communication between facility-based providers and hospital-based infectious disease consultants. However, facility-based clinicians must be aware of the limited level of care that can be provided in an infirmary.[53] Any patient with evidence of sepsis or who is suspected or found to have active bacteremia should be transferred to an emergency department immediately for further evaluation. If a patient is unstable, blood cultures can be drawn, and an initial dose of antibiotics administered on site while arranging transfer, but diligence in timely communicating microbiologic results to hospital-based care teams is critically important.

Chronic Infections

Apart from differences in the delivery system, managing HIV in correctional settings is not substantially different from doing so in the community (see **Fig. 2**).[54] Policies regarding HIV screening vary according to jurisdiction but universal opt-out screening on intake is recommended by the US Centers for Disease Control and Prevention for all jails and prisons (see **Table 1**) and is increasingly being implemented.[55,56] Universal screening in jails is somewhat more challenging than in prisons or community supervision agencies, owing to high turnover of individuals being admitted for stays of only a few days. Nearly all prisons and jails offer HIV testing in some circumstance, but in 1 survey, only 56% of prisons reported providing routine HIV screening at intake (including both opt-in and opt-out), whereas only 4% of jails provided routine screening.[56]

Once HIV is detected, either through screening or self-report, all incarcerated individuals with HIV in the United States should have access to safe and effective first-line antiretroviral (ARV) regimens, with regular monitoring of viral load and CD4$^+$ T-cell counts, vaccinations, and any indicated prophylaxis against opportunistic infections. However, limited data exist to assess how consistently these measures are available.[54] Many state prison systems fund ARV provision through the 340b funding mechanism,[57] avoiding the cost control hurdles (eg, prior authorization) of health insurance plans in the community. Although correctional health systems can generally provide consistent ARV access through established pharmacy relationships, interruptions can occur during transfers between institutions or trips to local courts for judicial proceedings. Health care providers responsible for HIV care in criminal justice settings must ensure adequate protocols are in place to prepare nursing and pharmacy staff for such events.

A substantial proportion of people living with HIV/AIDS in correctional institutions were not engaged in HIV care before arrest.[58] For these individuals, arrest and subsequent incarceration therefore represents an opportunity for engagement or reengagement with ARV therapy and other indicated preventive measures. As a consequence, providers of HIV care in correctional settings must be vigilant for signs of immune reconstitution inflammatory syndrome. People living with HIV/AIDS have relatively consistent access to ARVs while incarcerated, and adherence can be enhanced by administering ARVs under daily direct observation if requested by a provider. As a result, for people living with HIV/AIDS with criminal justice involvement, rates of retention in HIV care and viral suppression during incarceration are significantly higher than in the community (**Fig. 4**).[58]

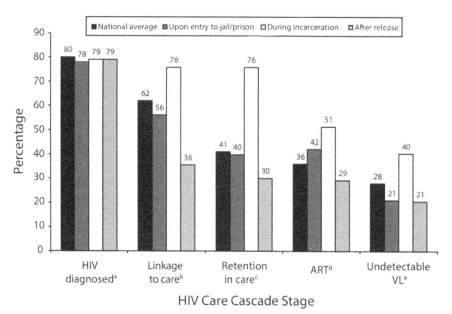

Fig. 4. Care cascade for HIV before, during, and after incarceration. (*From* Iroh PA., Mayo H., Nijhawan AE. The HIV Care Cascade Before, During, and After Incarceration: A Systematic Review and Data Synthesis. American Journal of Public Health 2015;105(7):e5–16; with permission.)

Unfortunately, however, the stability in HIV virologic control associated with incarceration proves fragile, and rates of viral suppression return to prearrest levels after release.[58] Individuals reentering the community from jail or prison face a number of complex and simultaneous challenges, including establishing stable housing, finding employment, reconnecting with friends and loved ones, and meeting requirements for parole, all while reengaging with community-based medical providers, and reactivating or reenrolling in health insurance coverage.[59–61] These competing demands can provoke anxiety, exacerbating the cue-associated cravings that are often stimulated by returning to prior settings of substance use. Furthermore, the lack of patient autonomy in correctional settings can, in our experience, create a dependence on institutional support (eg, directly observed medication administration) that is not available in the community. Thus, interruptions in ARV coverage are common after release from incarceration. In a landmark study of people living with HIV/AIDS being released from the state prison system in Texas during the period of 2004 to 2007, only 5.4% of patients succeeded in filling an ARV prescription within the first 10 days of release and 30.0% within 60 days.[62] Enrolling in an AIDS Drug Assistance Program before release can decrease the chance of treatment interruption.

Peer navigation has emerged as one of the most effective interventions to improve retention in HIV care and ARV adherence upon release.[63] In a large randomized trial of a structured, 12-session behavioral intervention administered by a peer-navigator among HIV-positive patients being released from the Los Angeles County Jail, viral suppression was maintained in 49.6% of patients receiving the intervention, compared with 36% of controls who receiving standard transitional case management alone.[64] Of note, the intervention was equally effective in people who use substances and those who did not.[64] Similar outcomes have been reported among HIV-positive patients receiving care in specialized "transitions clinics," which integrate peer navigators with lived experience of the criminal justice system into comprehensive, patient-centered primary care.[61] However, peer navigation services are available in only a select few jurisdictions and community clinics around the United States. The Centers for Disease Control and Prevention recommends that, before release, correctional facilities make an appointment with a community health care provider, assist with enrollment in an entitlement program, and provide a copy of the medical record and a supply of HIV medications.[55] Advocating for correctional systems to suspend, rather than terminate Medicaid enrollment for individuals on intake can also decrease interruptions in HIV care.[65]

Chronic HCV infection is substantially more prevalent than HIV, but screening for HCV is less common and access to treatment is currently very limited.[66] The prevalence of HCV varies regionally, but estimates range between 40% and 80% among people who inject drugs.[67,68] In state prison populations, HCV seroprevalence estimates range from 6% in Idaho to 40% in New Mexico.[66] Novel direct-acting antiviral therapies are well-tolerated and highly effective, but their cost is limiting or prohibitive for most correctional health systems (even if cost effective for society as a whole).[69] As the cost of treatment begins to decrease with competition from newer treatment options, HCV treatment in jails and prisons is rapidly expanding.[70] Following guidelines from the Federal Bureau of Prisons, direct-acting antiviral therapy is often prioritized for patients with higher degrees of hepatic fibrosis owing to resource constraints.[71] The degree of fibrosis can be assessed with easy to calculate clinical scores, such as the AST to Platelet Ratio Index or Fibrosis-4 score, or with more costly—but more precise—noninvasive measures such as transient elastography and direct biomarkers when available. Given the expense of the medications, administering them as directly observed therapy is reasonable and may improve adherence.[72]

Treatment outcomes in correctional settings are comparable with published results from community treatment programs with reported rates of sustained viral response generally greater than 90%.[70,73] However, release from incarceration or transfer to another correctional facility before completion of direct-acting antiviral therapy remains a barrier to successful treatment.[70] As with HIV, postrelease linkage to care for HCV is challenging and marked by high rates of loss to follow-up.[70,74] Early studies of peer navigation for HCV treatment after release from incarceration have been less promising than with HIV[74] and, given these challenges, universal HCV screening at intake to correctional facilities remains relatively low.[75] However, expanded screening may be on the horizon, given the recent recommendation by the US Preventive Services Task Force that all adults be screened for HCV regardless of age or known risk factors.[76]

OPPORTUNITIES FOR PREVENTIVE CARE

Although it may have deleterious effects for individuals who are already made vulnerable by overlapping social and structural factors, an episode of criminal justice involvement also presents an opportunity to provide preventive health needs that are often underutilized by people with OUD and other SUDs (see **Table 1**). The Centers for Disease Control and Prevention guidelines recommend screening all people who inject drugs for sexually transmitted infections, HIV, chronic hepatitis B virus, chronic HCV, and latent tuberculosis infection.[77] Universal screening for latent tuberculosis infection with either tuberculin skin testing or IFN-gamma release assays on intake is standard in most correctional facilities.[78] All people with OUD who are not known to be either immune or actively infected should be vaccinated against hepatitis A and hepatitis B. All people with OUD who are hepatitis B surface antibody negative and not found to have evidence of chronic hepatitis B virus infection should receive vaccination, including individuals with isolated hepatitis B core antibody who remain at risk of infection. Up-to-date booster dosing with tetanus and diphtheria toxoids every 10 years should be maintained for all incarcerated adults,[79] and people who inject drugs are at increased risk of exposure to tetanus.

Patient-Centered Care

Owing to the fear of criminal sanctions for ongoing opioid use and widespread stigma experienced by people who use drugs in health care and criminal justice settings, patients with OUD may exhibit substantial mistrust toward medical providers.[80,81] Approaching a patient with warmth, asking about their substance use in a nonjudgmental fashion, and reinforcing protections for the confidentiality of health information may help to overcome these barriers and facilitate meaningful engagement. Formal harm reduction services (eg, syringe exchange, condom distribution, etc.) may be limited in correctional settings, but taking a harm reduction approach is possible with any patient (see **Table 1**). The provision of trauma-informed care is another key principle guiding health care engagement for patients with OUD. Trauma and post-traumatic stress disorder are highly prevalent among people with addiction,[17] as well as those with criminal justice involvement.[15,82] Training staff to recognize and deescalate behavioral manifestations of trauma-related psychological symptoms can promote a health care environment that emphasizes safety and trust.[83] Ultimately, providing comprehensive, patient-centered care for people with OUD in settings of incarceration requires a willingness to promote health within a system defined by deprivation and advocate for the community standard of care (see **Figs. 1** and **2**).

DISCLOSURE

The authors have no conflicts of interest to disclose. This work was supported in part by grants from the National Institute of Mental Health [T32 MH 019139–30] to D. Winetsky and from the National Institute on Drug Abuse [R34 DA 045592] to A. Nijhawan.

REFERENCES

1. Longo DL, Compton WM, Jones CM, et al. Relationship between Nonmedical Prescription-Opioid Use and Heroin Use. N Engl J Med 2016;374(2):154–63.
2. NIDA Overdose Death Rates. National Institute on Drug Abuse. Available at: NIDA. "Overdose Death Rates." National Institute on Drug Abuse. Available at: https://www.drugabuse.gov/related-topics/trends-statistics/overdose-death-rates. Accessed December 10, 2019.
3. Centers for Disease Control and Prevention (CDC). HIV and AIDS–United States, 1981-2000. MMWR Morb Mortal Wkly Rep 2001;50(21):430–4.
4. Scholl L, Seth P, Kariisa M, et al. Drug and Opioid-Involved Overdose Deaths — United States, 2013–2017. MMWR Morb Mortal Wkly Rep 2018;67(5152).
5. Zibbell JE, Asher AK, Patel RC, et al. Increases in Acute Hepatitis C Virus Infection Related to a Growing Opioid Epidemic and Associated Injection Drug Use, United States, 2004 to 2014. Am J Public Health 2018;108(2):175–81.
6. Schranz AJ, Fleischauer A, Chu VH, et al. Trends in drug use-associated infective endocarditis and heart valve surgery, 2007 to 2017: a study of statewide discharge data. Ann Intern Med 2019;170(1):31–40.
7. Szalavitz M. What the media gets wrong about opioids. Columbia Journalism Review 2018.

8. Brico E. A dangerous fentanyl myth lives on. Columbia Journalism Review 2019.

9. Winkelman TNA, Chang VW, Binswanger IA. Health, Polysubstance Use, and Criminal Justice Involvement Among Adults With Varying Levels of Opioid Use. JAMA Netw Open 2018;1(3):e180558.

10. Han B, Compton WM, Blanco C, et al. Prescription Opioid Use, Misuse, and Use Disorders in U.S. Adults: 2015 National Survey on Drug Use and Health. Ann Intern Med 2017;167(5):293–301.

11. Kaeble D, Cowhig M. Correctional populations in the United States, 2016. Washington, DC: Bureau of Justice Statistics, United States Department of Justice; 2018. p. 14.

12. Bureau of Justice Statistics of the United States Department of Justice. Criminal Justice System Description. Available at: https://www.bjs.gov/content/justsys.cfm. Accessed December 20, 2019.

13. Maruschak LM, Berzofsky M. Medical problems of state and federal prisoners and jail inmates, 2011-12. Washington, DC: Bureau of Justice Statistics, United States Department of Justice; 2015.

14. CASA Columbia behind bars II: substance abuse and America's prison population. New York: The National Center on Addiction and Substance Abuse at Columbia University; 2010.

15. Wolff N, Huening J, Shi J, et al. Trauma exposure and posttraumatic stress disorder among incarcerated men. J Urban Health 2014;91(4):707–19.

16. Rold WJ. Thirty years after Estelle v. Gamble: a legal retrospective. J Correct Health Care 2008;14(1):11–20.

17. Singer M. A dose of drugs, a touch of violence, a case of AIDS: conceptualizing the SAVA syndemic. Free Inq Creat Sociol 1996;24(2):99–110.

18. Binswanger IA, Blatchford PJ, Mueller SR, et al. Mortality after prison release: opioid overdose and other causes of death, risk factors, and time trends from 1999 to 2009. Ann Intern Med 2013;159(9):592.

19. Wood E, Li K, Small W, et al. Recent incarceration independently associated with syringe sharing by injection drug users. Public Health Reports 2005;120(2):150–6.

20. Stone J, Fraser H, Lim AG, et al. Incarceration history and risk of HIV and hepatitis C virus acquisition among people who inject drugs: a systematic review and meta-analysis. Lancet Infect Dis 2018;18(12):1397–409.

21. Allen SA, Aburabi R. When security and medicine missions conflict: confidentiality in prison settings. Int J Prison Health 2016;12(2):73–7.

22. Rappaport ES, Reynolds HN, Baucom S, et al. Telehealth support of managed care for a correctional system: the open architecture telehealth model. Telemed J E Health 2018;24(1):54–60.

23. Glowa-Kollisch S, Graves J, Dickey N, et al. Data-driven human rights: using dual loyalty trainings to promote the care of vulnerable patients in jail. Health Hum Rights 2015;17(1):124.

24. Nunn A, Zaller N, Dickman S, et al. Methadone and buprenorphine prescribing and referral practices in US prison systems: results from a nationwide survey. Drug Alcohol Depend 2009;105(1–2):83–8.

25. Friedmann PD, Hoskinson R, Gordon M, et al. Medication-assisted treatment in criminal justice agencies affiliated with the Criminal Justice-Drug Abuse Treatment Studies (CJ-DATS): availability, barriers, and intentions. Substance Abuse 2012;33(1):9–18.

26. Comer S, Cunningham C, Fishman MJ, et al. National practice guideline for the use of medications in the treatment of addiction involving opioid use. Rockville (MD): American Society of Addiction Medicine; 2015.
27. Taylor K. Jail Ordered to Give Inmate Methadone for Opioid Addiction in Far-Reaching Ruling. New York Times 2018.
28. Wickersham JA, Azar MM, Cannon CM, et al. Validation of a brief measure of opioid dependence: the Rapid Opioid Dependence Screen (RODS). J Correct Health Care 2015;21(1):12–26.
29. Clarke JG, Martin RA, Gresko SA, et al. The first comprehensive program for opioid use disorder in a US statewide correctional system. Am J Public Health 2018;108(10):1323–5.
30. Rich JD, McKenzie M, Larney S, et al. Methadone continuation versus forced withdrawal on incarceration in a combined US prison and jail: a randomised, open-label trial. Lancet 2015;386(9991):350–9.
31. Hedrich D, Alves P, Farrell M, et al. The effectiveness of opioid maintenance treatment in prison settings: a systematic review: opioid maintenance in prison. Addiction 2012;107(3):501–17.
32. Brinkley-Rubinstein L, Peterson M, Clarke J, et al. The benefits and implementation challenges of the first state-wide comprehensive medication for addictions program in a unified jail and prison setting. Drug Alcohol Depend 2019;205: 107514.
33. Green TC, Clarke J, Brinkley-Rubinstein L, et al. Postincarceration Fatal Overdoses After Implementing Medications for Addiction Treatment in a Statewide Correctional System. JAMA Psychiatry 2018;75(4):405.
34. Committee on Medication-Assisted Treatment for Opioid Use Disorder, Board on Health Sciences Policy, Health and Medicine Division, et al. Medications for opioid use disorder save lives. Washington, DC: National Academies Press; 2019.
35. Strang J. Loss of tolerance and overdose mortality after inpatient opiate detoxification: follow up study. BMJ 2003;326(7396):959–60.
36. Haber PS, Demirkol A, Lange K, et al. Management of injecting drug users admitted to hospital. Lancet 2009;374(9697):1284–93.
37. Maradiaga JA, Nahvi S, Cunningham CO, et al. "I Kicked the Hard Way. I Got Incarcerated." Withdrawal from Methadone During Incarceration and Subsequent Aversion to Medication Assisted Treatments. J Subst Abuse Treat 2016; 62:49–54.
38. Mitchell SG, Kelly SM, Brown BS, et al. Incarceration and opioid withdrawal: the experiences of methadone patients and out-of-treatment heroin users. J Psychoactive Drugs 2009;41(2):145–52.
39. Gordon MS, Kinlock TW, Schwartz RP, et al. A randomized clinical trial of methadone maintenance for prisoners: findings at 6 months post-release. Addiction 2008;103(8):1333–42.
40. Lee JD, Friedmann PD, Kinlock TW, et al. Extended-Release Naltrexone to Prevent Opioid Relapse in Criminal Justice Offenders. N Engl J Med 2016; 374(13):1232–42.
41. Aloe J. Vermont prison staff will carry opioid rescue medication Narcan after rise in overdoses. Burlington Free Press. Available at: https://www.burlingtonfreepress.com/story/news/2019/01/22/vermont-prisons-expand-access-overdose-reversal-drug-naloxone/2579110002/. Accessed December 17, 2019.
42. Zucker H, Annucci AJ, Stancliff S, et al. Overdose prevention for prisoners in New York: a novel program and collaboration. Harm Reduct J 2015;12(1):51.

43. Goodnough A, Zernike K. Seizing on Opioid Crisis, a Drug Maker Lobbies Hard for Its Product. New York Times 2017.
44. Larochelle MR, Bernson D, Land T, et al. Medication for opioid use disorder after nonfatal opioid overdose and association with mortality: a cohort study. Ann Intern Med 2018;169(3):137.
45. Binswanger IA, Glanz JM. Potential risk window for opioid overdose related to treatment with extended-release injectable naltrexone. Drug Saf 2018;41(10): 979–80.
46. Gordon MS, Kinlock TW, Schwartz RP, et al. Buprenorphine Treatment for Probationers and Parolees. Substance Abuse 2015;36(2):217–25.
47. Springer SA, Qiu J, Saber-Tehrani AS, et al. Retention on Buprenorphine Is Associated with High Levels of Maximal Viral Suppression among HIV-Infected Opioid Dependent Released Prisoners. PLoS One 2012;7(5):e38335.
48. Springer SA, Korthuis PT, Del Rio C. Integrating treatment at the intersection of opioid use disorder and infectious disease epidemics in medical settings: a call for action after a National Academies of Sciences, Engineering, and Medicine Workshop. Ann Intern Med 2018;169(5):335–6.
49. Young JD, Patel M, Badowski M, et al. Improved virologic suppression with HIV subspecialty care in a large prison system using telemedicine: an observational study with historical controls. Clin Infect Dis 2014;59(1):123–6.
50. Arora S, Thornton K, Jenkusky SM, et al. Project ECHO: linking university specialists with rural and prison-based clinicians to improve care for people with chronic hepatitis C in New Mexico. Public Health Reports 2007;122(Suppl 2):74–7.
51. Moazen B, Saeedi Moghaddam S, Silbernagl MA, et al. Prevalence of Drug Injection, Sexual Activity, Tattooing, and Piercing Among Prison Inmates. Epidemiol Rev 2018;40(1):58–69.
52. Paladino JA, Poretz D. Outpatient parenteral antimicrobial therapy today. Clin Infect Dis 2010;51(Suppl 2):S198–208.
53. Paris JE. Infirmary care. Correctional medicine. St. Louis (MO): Mosby; 1998. p. 77–85.
54. Springer SA, Altice FL. Managing HIV/AIDS in correctional settings. Curr HIV/ AIDS Rep 2005;2(4):165–70.
55. Beckwith C, Bick J, Chow W, et al. HIV testing implementation guidance for correctional settings. Atlanta (GA): Centers for Disease Control and Prevention; 2009.
56. Solomon L, Montague BT, Beckwith CG, et al. Survey Finds That Many Prisons And Jails Have Room To Improve HIV Testing And Coordination Of Postrelease Treatment. Health Aff 2014;33(3):434–42.
57. Huh K, Boucher A, McGaffey F, et al. Pharmaceuticals in State Prisons: how departments of corrections purchase, use and monitor prescription drugs. Philadelphia: The Pew Charitable Trusts; 2017.
58. Iroh PA, Mayo H, Nijhawan AE. The HIV care cascade before, during, and after incarceration: a systematic review and data synthesis. Am J Public Health 2015;105(7):e5–16.
59. van Olphen J, Freudenberg N, Fortin P, et al. Community reentry: perceptions of people with substance use problems returning home from New York City Jails. J Urban Health 2006;83(3):372–81.
60. Visher C, LaVigne N, Travis J. Returning home: understanding the challenges of prisoner reentry: Maryland Pilot Study: findings from Baltimore. Washington, DC: Urban Institute, Justice Policy Center; 2004.

61. Masyukova MI, Hanna DB, Fox AD. HIV treatment outcomes among formerly incarcerated transitions clinic patients in a high prevalence setting. Health Justice 2018;6(1):16.

62. Baillargeon J, Giordano TP, Rich JD, et al. Accessing antiretroviral therapy following release from prison. JAMA 2009;301(8):848.

63. Westergaard RP, Hochstatter KR, Andrews PN, et al. Effect of patient navigation on transitions of HIV care after release from prison: a retrospective cohort study. AIDS Behav 2019;23(9):2549–57.

64. Cunningham WE, Weiss RE, Nakazono T, et al. Effectiveness of a peer navigation intervention to sustain viral suppression among HIV-positive men and transgender women released from jail: the LINK LA Randomized Clinical Trial. JAMA Intern Med 2018;178(4):542.

65. Boutwell AE, Freedman J. Coverage expansion and the criminal justice-involved population: implications for plans and service connectivity. Health Aff (Millwood) 2014;33(3):482–6.

66. Spaulding AC, Anderson EJ, Khan MA, et al. HIV and HCV in U.S. Prisons and jails: the correctional facility as a bellwether over time for the community's infections. AIDSRev 2017;19(3):301.

67. Lelutiu-Weinberger C, Pouget ER, Des Jarlais DDC, et al. A meta-analysis of the hepatitis C virus distribution in diverse racial/ethnic drug injector groups. Soc Sci Med 2009;68(3):579–90.

68. Des Jarlais DC, Arasteh K, Feelemyer J, et al. Hepatitis C virus prevalence and estimated incidence among new injectors during the opioid epidemic in New York City, 2000–2017: protective effects of non-injecting drug use. Drug Alcohol Depend 2018;192:74–9.

69. Nguyen JT, Rich JD, Brockmann BW, et al. A budget impact analysis of newly available hepatitis C therapeutics and the financial burden on a state correctional system. J Urban Health 2015;92(4):635–49.

70. Chan J. Outcomes of hepatitis C virus treatment in a jail population: successes and challenges facing Expansion. Las Vegas (NV): 2019.

71. Federal Bureau of prisons evaluation and management of chronic hepatitis C virus (HCV) infection. Washington, DC: Federal Bureau of Prisons; 2018.

72. McDermott CL, Lockhart CM, Devine B. Outpatient directly observed therapy for hepatitis C among people who use drugs: a systematic review and meta-analysis. J Virus Erad 2018;4(2):118–22.

73. Sterling RK, Cherian R, Lewis S, et al. Treatment of HCV in the Department of Corrections in the Era of Oral Medications. J Correct Health Care 2018;24(2):127–36.

74. Akiyama MJ, Columbus D, MacDonald R, et al. Linkage to hepatitis C care after incarceration in jail: a prospective, single arm clinical trial. BMC Infect Dis 2019;19(1):703.

75. Spaulding A, Chhatwal J, Thanthong-Knight S, et al. HepCorrections. Available at: http://www.hepcorrections.org/. Accessed December 18, 2019.

76. United States Preventive Services Task Force Draft Recommendation Statement. Hepatitis C virus infection in adolescents and adults: screening - US Preventive Services Task Force. Available at: https://www.uspreventiveservicestaskforce.org/Page/Document/draft-recommendation-statement/hepatitis-c-screening1. Accessed January 14, 2020.

77. Centers for Disease Control and Prevention (CDC). Integrated prevention services for HIV infection, viral hepatitis, sexually transmitted diseases, and tuberculosis for persons who use drugs illicitly: summary guidance from CDC and the

U.S. Department of Health and Human Services. MMWR Recomm Rep 2012; 61(RR-5):1–40.

78. Nijhawan AE, Iroh PA, Brown LS, et al. Cost analysis of tuberculin skin test and the QuantiFERON-TB Gold In-tube test for tuberculosis screening in a correctional setting in Dallas, Texas, USA. BMC Infect Dis 2016;16(1):564.

79. Liang JL, Tiwari T, Moro P, et al. Prevention of pertussis, tetanus, and diphtheria with vaccines in the United States: recommendations of the Advisory Committee on Immunization Practices (ACIP). MMWR Recomm Rep 2018;67(2):1–44.

80. McNeil R, Small W, Wood E, et al. Hospitals as a "risk environment": an ethno-epidemiological study of voluntary and involuntary discharge from hospital against medical advice among people who inject drugs. Soc Sci Med 2014; 105:59–66.

81. Paquette CE, Syvertsen JL, Pollini RA. Stigma at every turn: health services experiences among people who inject drugs. International J Drug Policy 2018;57: 104–10.

82. Jäggi LJ, Mezuk B, Watkins DC, et al. The relationship between trauma, arrest, and incarceration History among Black Americans: findings from the National Survey of American Life. Soc Ment Health 2016;6(3):187–206.

83. Chaudhri S, Zweig KC, Hebbar P, et al. Trauma-informed care: a strategy to improve primary healthcare engagement for persons with criminal justice system involvement. J Gen Intern Med 2019;34(6):1048–52.

84. Centers for Disease Control and Prevention (CDC), National Center for HIV/AIDS, Viral Hepatitis, STD, and TB Prevention. Prevention and control of tuberculosis in correctional and detention facilities: recommendations from CDC. Endorsed by the Advisory Council for the Elimination of Tuberculosis, the National Commission on Correctional Health Care, and the American Correctional Association. MMWR Recomm Rep 2006;55(RR-9):1–44.

Harm Reduction Services to Prevent and Treat Infectious Diseases in People Who Use Drugs

Kinna Thakarar, DO, MPH[a,*], Katherine Nenninger, MD[b],
Wollelaw Agmas, MD[c]

KEYWORDS

- Harm reduction • Preventive health services • Social justice
- People who inject drugs • PWID

KEY POINTS

- Harm reduction is a social justice movement and encompasses nonjudgmental strategies to mitigate negative consequences from ongoing drug use.
- Syringe service programs and supervised infection facilities are evidence-based strategies to prevent injection drug use-associated infections and overdoses.
- Clinicians can integrate harm reduction strategies into their practice and work with community partners to advocate for the health and safety of people who inject drugs.

WHAT IS HARM REDUCTION?

Harm reduction encompasses practical strategies, programs, and policies to help mitigate the negative consequences of drug use. Grounded in social justice, harm reduction is based on several principles and includes treating people who use drugs with respect and compassion. Harm reduction is a pragmatic approach where providers can offer people a range of options to reduce harm and individualize care plans to protect their health, while respecting the autonomy of people who use drugs.[1]

This work was supported by grant U54 GM115516 from the National Institutes of Health for the Northern New England Clinical and Translational Research network.

[a] Infectious Disease and Addiction Medicine, Maine Medical Center/Tufts University School of Medicine, 50 Foden Road, South Portland, ME 04106, USA; [b] Preventive Medicine, Maine Medical Center/Tufts University School of Medicine, 22 Bramhall Street, Portland, ME 04102, USA; [c] Infectious Disease, Maine Medical Center/Tufts University School of Medicine, 22 Bramhall Street, Portland, ME 04102, USA
* Corresponding author. 41 Donald Bean Drive, Suite B, South Portland, ME 04106.
E-mail address: kthakarar@mmc.org

SYRINGE SERVICE PROGRAMS

The term "syringe service program" (SSP), also referred to as "needle exchanges" or "needle and syringe programs," is inclusive of any setting that provides needles, syringes, and other supplies intended for injection of drugs.[2] SSPs were first established in Europe in the 1980s during the human immunodeficiency virus (HIV)/AIDS epidemic.[3] Since then, as evidence has mounted supporting their value, SSPs have been implemented worldwide.[4]

Most SSPs offer free or low-cost harm reduction services such naloxone rescue kits, education, infectious disease screening and vaccination, wound care, and recovery resources.[5–7] Identifying and screening for infectious diseases at SSPs or through SSP outreach work has resulted in successful linkage to care.[8] Onsite clinical care for HIV and hepatitis C (HCV) is less common, but can exist.[9] Since many people who inject drugs (PWID) avoid health care settings, but may be willing to engage with SSPs, integrated testing and outreach has strong potential to identify otherwise undiagnosed infectious diseases.[7] Mobile SSP units, based out of vehicles that can travel to several locations, are also poised to further geographically expand screening.[2]

In the United States, the political and funding environment for SSPs has been largely unfavorable, although recent high-profile HIV outbreaks have spurred some policy changes.[10,11] Services vary significantly in scope and scale and are often limited by regulations and funding.[12–15] Policy needs to evolve to allow for expansion, innovation, and research on SSP delivery models such as mobile delivery models and peer sharing networks.[6]

Evidence of Syringe Service Programs Benefit in Infectious Disease Prevention

A critical component of SSPs is the promotion of safe injection practices through supply distribution and education. An understanding of these supplies, their proper use,

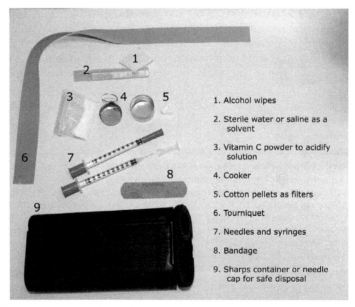

1. Alcohol wipes

2. Sterile water or saline as a solvent

3. Vitamin C powder to acidify solution

4. Cooker

5. Cotton pellets as filters

6. Tourniquet

7. Needles and syringes

8. Bandage

9. Sharps container or needle cap for safe disposal

Fig. 1. Drug preparation equipment.

Table 1
Summary of equipment for drug preparation process

Street Examples[95]	Recommended Supplies	Purpose[96–104]
No skin cleanser, tap water, soap and water, hand sanitizer, cloth/tissue, alcoholic beverage	Alcohol wipes	Clean hands and skin at injection site before injection
Spoons, bottle caps	Cookers	Sterile metal cup in which to heat up/dissolve drug powder into solvent
Tap or bottle water, pond or puddle water, spit, toilet water	Sterile water or saline	Solvent for drug solution
Lemon juice, vinegar, kettle descaler	Vitamin C	Acidify solution to help dissolve crack cocaine and "black tar" heroin
Cigarettes, cotton balls, cotton tipped swabs, tampons, lint	Dental/cotton pellets	Catch particulates as the drug solution is drawn up into the syringe; can decrease bacterial loads
Reused needles	New needles	Injecting into vein
Socks, belts, gloves, condoms	Tourniquets	Prepare vein for injection
Reused syringes	Syringes	Injecting into vein
Reused needles/syringes, trash, street	Sharps containers	Safe storage, return syringes and needles to SSP for exchange if available
No wound care	Wound care supplies: band-aids, gauze, gloves, bandage wraps, tape, ointments	Protect open wounds
No preventive services	Fentanyl test strips, condoms, naloxone kits, PrEP	Reduce overdoses, reduce sexually transmitted infections

Abbreviation: PrEP, pre-exposure prophylaxis for HIV prevention.

and risk reduction is important for communicating effectively with PWID. Items that may be available at SSPs are shown in **Fig. 1** and are summarized in **Table 1**.

Although it can be challenging to study the effect of SSPs in the real-world setting, SSPs have clearly reduced high-risk injection behaviors such as equipment sharing, reuse, and high injection frequency.[15] This risk reduction can extend beyond SSP users to their peer network.

In terms of injection drug use (IDU)-associated infections, there is strong evidence that SSPs decrease HIV and its associated costs.[15,16] Implementation of SSPs in conjunction with other harm reduction measures in the midst of HIV outbreaks have proven effective measures to curb ongoing transmission.[17] Although pre-exposure prophylaxis (PrEP) for HIV prevention uptake has been low among PWID, SSPs can be a channel for increasing PrEP awareness and use[18]

The quality of evidence is more limited than for HIV, but SSPs can also potentially play a role in decreasing other IDU-associated infections. HCV can remain on drug equipment surfaces for several days; not surprisingly, because they distribute clean equipment, SSPs can decrease HCV risk.[19,20] Distance from SSP can increase HCV risk, whereas frequent SSP use decreases HCV risk.[21,22] Although not well-studied, infrequent SSP use has been linked to HBV.[16,23] Additionally, decreasing injection risk behaviors among SSP users suggests promise in reducing skin and soft tissue infections (SSTI), which are prevalent among PWID.[7]

Regulations Surrounding Syringe Service Programs in the United States

Despite the proven and potential benefits, SSPs remain somewhat controversial in the United States owing to the "war on drugs" ideology and the misconception that substance use disorders (SUD) represent a moral failing, as well as the fear that SSPs might lead to drug use initiation.[10,24] At the time of inaugural SSP development in the 1980s, one notable barrier was the 1988 ban on the use of federal funding for SSP programs until they could be proven safe and effective.[10,24]

As evidence on the benefits of SSPs mounted, over the decades there were several attempts to lift the funding ban.[24] After the HIV outbreak in Scott County, Indiana, brought national attention to the event and SSPs were included in the public health response, the federal ban was removed again in 2015 to allow for the use of federal funds to support SSP operations in areas or jurisdictions deemed at risk for outbreaks, excepting the actual purchase of needles and syringes.[10] This change has facilitated SSP expansion.[25] However, SSPs have been slow to spread to vulnerable areas, reflecting continuing stigma as well as hurdles posed by state and local drug paraphernalia laws.[26] By 2015, many states had updated policies to allow for licensed SSPs, but today there are still several states that prohibit them.[11] Other regulations also affect the number of syringes that can be distributed or exchanged, for example, requiring a used syringe to be collected for each clean syringe dispensed (ie, 1-for-1 syringe exchange).[27] Overall, in the United States there continues to be a complicated regulatory landscape that hinders adequate access to sterile injection supplies.

In contrast, other countries including Canada, Australia, and many European Union nations are permissive and supportive of SSPs, with costs shared by national and local governments and even international organizations.[4,28] Many countries have also explored the use of safe injection facilities, which is discussed further in the next section.

Summary

- SSPs can decrease IDU-associated infections
- SSPs vary in availability of preventative services, such as vaccinations and PrEP, however PWID have shown interest in these important services.
- Despite evidence showing the benefits of SSPs, in the United States several regulatory barriers exist that prevent SSP expansion

SUPERVISED INJECTION FACILITIES

Individuals can bring preowned drugs to supervised injection facilities (SIFs), which are safe environments to inject drugs. SIFs are also sometimes referred to as medically supervised injection centers, safe injection facilities, supervised consumption facilities, drug consumption rooms, or overdose prevention sites. Facility staff members do not directly assist in injecting or handling any drugs preowned by the individual, but they are present to provide sterile injection equipment, answer questions on safe injection techniques, administer first aid when needed, and monitor for overdose.

SIFs were first started in the 1970s and have been operating in Europe, Australia, and Canada for decades,[29] but no legally authorized facilities exist in the United States to date. Insite, the first SIF in North America, was opened in Vancouver, Canada in 2003, as a response to the devastating epidemics of HIV and drug overdose deaths and was legally sanctioned in 2011. Mobile and in-hospital SIFs also exist in some countries.[30,31] In the United States, SIFs have faced opposition; however, SIFs in Canada and Australia have undergone numerous evaluations showing that they have multiple health and community benefits.[32,33] SIF benefits and barriers are discussed further in this section.[33–38]

Benefits of Supervised Injection Facilities

Reduce morbidity and mortality
A cohort study that compared mortality before and after Insite was opened in Vancouver, British Columbia, showed a decrease in overdose death by 35%.[34] Another study found that the number of deaths averted by Insite ranged from 1.9 to 11.7 deaths per year.[35] SIFs have reported thousands of witnessed overdoses; however, no deaths have been reported thus far.[37,39] Notably, a study from Sydney, Australia, also reported a 67% decrease in the number of ambulance calls for overdose reversal in a SIF neighborhood.[36,39]

Reduce infections
In addition to monitoring for overdoses, SIFs provide clients education on safe injection techniques, provide vaccinations, and conduct screening and treatment for sexually transmitted infections.[40] PWID who use SIFs frequently practice safer injection, and there have been significant decreases in prolonged hospitalizations for IDU-associated infections.[41,42] Modeling studies have shown that SIFs can decrease incident HIV and HCV infections[43] and the costs incurred to provide lifelong HIV care and expensive HCV treatment.[37,38,41,42,44–46]

Reduce cost
Studies have shown that SIFs are cost effective. One cost-effectiveness analysis showed that a SIF was associated with an incremental net savings of almost $14 million and 920 life-years gained over a 10-year period.[43] There are expected cost savings from averted HIV and HCV, decreased skin and soft tissue infections, averted overdose deaths, and increased uptake of medications for opioid use disorder (MOUD).[43,45–48]

Reduce drug use and increase treatment uptake
Studies in Vancouver have shown that SIF users reported less frequent reuse of syringes, and in 1 study, 57% of clients entered MOUD treatment programs.[49,50] SIFs can also facilitate referrals to the hospital for earlier intervention.[41,42]

Decrease public injecting and increase public safety
Observational studies have reported beneficial effects of SIFs for PWID and neighborhoods. PWID who used SIFs are less likely to report needle sharing (71%), to dispose of syringes unsafely (56%), and to inject in public places. By decreasing fatal drug overdoses in the streets and reducing public drug use, public safety is maintained.[37,50–52]

Barriers to Safe Injection Facilities

The barriers to opening SIFs in the United States arise from the public and legal issues that are presented in **Tables 2** and **3**. SIF opponents report concerns that SIFs are

Table 2
Supervised injection facilities in the United States

Barriers	Arguments and Evidence to Support SIFs
Legal: Legality complicated owing to federal and state government involvement. The US forbids: Possession of controlled substances Making places available for unlawful distribution or use of a controlled substance.[27]	CSA* meant to address drug purchasing and consumption (colloquially known as the "Crack House Statute")[27] CSA not meant to influence public health interventions/infringe on state public health authority[27]
Public opinion: Although evidence support SIFs, establishing SIFs can be challenging in the setting of public opposition	PWID need public support[98] SIFs are public health interventions that can reduce mortality, morbidity, and IDU-associated infections[37,44,48,99] SIFs reduce public injecting, crime and increase public safety[50–52]
Funding: SIFs may require significant startup and operating costs. Obtaining federal, state and local funding, in addition to outside donations, can be difficult owing to the legal controversies.	Cost saving[100,101] Life saving, lead to early medical interventions, and should be publicly funded[42]

Abbreviation: CSA, Controlled Substance Act.

morally or legally wrong and will promote drug use and increase crime rates; however, these fears are unsubstantiated.[33,53] In October 2019, a federal judge ruled that the bid of a nonprofit group, Safehouse, to open a SIF in Philadelphia did not violate federal law. Its opening, however, was halted in the setting of opposition.[54]

Summary

- SIFs are safe indoor spaces where PWID can inject their preowned drugs in the presence of trained staff
- SIFs decrease morbidity and mortality, while increasing treatment uptake and public safety
- The status of SIFs in the United States remains uncertain, although in 2019 a federal judge ruled that opening a SIF in Philadelphia would not violate federal law

INTEGRATING HARM REDUCTION INTO CLINICAL PRACTICE

Particularly in the setting of increasing stimulant use, harm reduction is an essential component to preventing IDU-associated infections. In addition to reviewing evidence-based harm reduction strategies to integrate into clinical practice, this section reviews the concept of low barrier programs and opportunities for providers to advocate for harm reduction policies.

Overdose Prevention

Naloxone is a cost-effective, rapidly acting opioid antagonist to reverse drug overdoses, and it is particularly effective when distributed directly to PWID.[55,56] In some states, standing orders for naloxone exist; that is, the ability for a person at risk of overdose and/or a potential bystander to purchase naloxone without a prescription.[57] Although anyone with prescribing authority is able to prescribe naloxone to patients

Table 3
Summary of drug preparation steps and safe injection counseling points

Drug Preparation Step	Counseling Points[69,70,102–106]
Injection site preparation	Wash hands before and after injection Use alcohol pads, gauze pads, and bandages at injection site Clean other surfaces blood may have touched (ie, tourniquets) To minimize SSTIs, avoid "skip popping" (injecting subcutaneously) or "muscle popping" (injecting intramuscularly) if unable to find veins Avoid major arteries and small veins Rotate injection sites
N/S	Avoid reusing N/S Although often done to recover residual drug, avoid licking needles If no clean N/S available, wash with full-strength bleach for >2 min
Filters	Cigarette or other filters that require manual manipulation increase infection risk Consider small, preformed pellets Use new filters with each injection
Cookers	Cooking drugs can decrease bacterial burden. Avoid reusing or sharing cookers
Dissolving drug	Use sterile water when possible
Acidifiers (used if injecting solids such as base heroin or crack cocaine)	Use vitamin C packets to minimize risk of fungal infections and vein damage Avoid excessive use (ie, entire vitamin C packet) owing to risk of vein damage Consider adding small amount of sodium bicarbonate to buffer solution at the end of drug preparation process[105]
Environment	Take your time; find a clean, safe space Avoid injecting alone To decrease overdose risk, inject yourself, rather than having someone else do it

Abbreviations: N/S, sterile needles and syringes; SSTIs, skin and soft tissue infections.

at risk for overdose, state laws vary in terms of prescriptions for third parties (ie, potential bystanders).[58]

Barriers to obtaining naloxone, such as stigma, inconvenience, cost, and lack of syringe service or community programs, have been reported.[58,59] Given these barriers, providers should prescribe naloxone. Despite its effectiveness, the uptake of prescribing naloxone has been suboptimal, often owing to a lack of provider training, lack of time, and/or concerns for "enabling" drug use.[60,61] Strategies to improve naloxone prescribing include partnering with community organizations who can deliver naloxone education to providers,[62,63] obtaining political and institutional support to streamline naloxone education and prescribing,[64,65] and the use of existing online resources (ie, naloxone training videos).[58,66] These strategies can help providers to improve their prescribing self-efficacy and to integrate naloxone prescribing into practice. In addition, providers should counsel patients on how to recognize the signs and symptoms of an overdose.

Counseling strategies to prevent overdoses are summarized in **Table 4**. In addition, fentanyl test strip technology, initially developed as a tool for detecting fentanyl in the

Table 4
Counseling points for overdose prevention

Mixing drugs	Use 1 drug at a time Minimize use of each drug Avoid mixing drugs with alcohol
Quality of drug	Test a small amount of drug first ("test shot") Purchase from same distributor Be cautious when switching between pills, know what you are using
Overdose plan	Do not use alone Keep door unlocked and/or slightly open Call a friend to check in Have naloxone ready
Mode of administration	Injecting and smoking increase overdose risk If using alone or concerns for decreased tolerance, snort if possible

From National Harm Reduction Coalition. Overdose Prevention Tips. Available at: https://harmreduction.org/wp-content/uploads/2012/11/HRC_ODprevention_worksheet9.pdf. Accessed March 2 2020; with permission.

urine, has been used by many PWID to detect fentanyl in their street drugs.[67] Although use of fentanyl test strips has been associated with overdose safety,[68] there are still some fentanyl test strip limitations, including an inability to quantify fentanyl and difficulty interpreting results.[67]

Safe Injection Techniques

Safe injection techniques can reduce complications from IDU-associated infections. Provider strategies to begin these discussions include: (1) an awareness of safe injection techniques, (2) a nonjudgmental manner, (3) an awareness of local resources and regulations (SSPs, mobile units, and local policies like pharmacist dispensing), and (4) the willingness to explore the patient barriers to accessing harm reduction services.

There are multiple steps in the drug preparation process, and specific counseling points for each step are summarized in **Table 3**.[69,70] Asking open-ended questions (eg, "Can you walk me through how you usually inject?") can help to begin these conversations. By understanding specific injection practices, providers can then make individualized suggestions to minimize infection risk.[71] Other factors, such as stigma and a lack of access to housing and/or SSPs or pharmacies may influence injection practices, so these issues should also be addressed.[72]

In Canada, providers have been successful in providing clean drug equipment for their patients; however, in the United States, state laws vary in terms of (1) possession of drug equipment, such as the number of needles/syringes an individual can carry and (2) provider ability to prescribe needles, syringes, and other supplies. Providers should also seek guidance from institutional or practice legal counsel to understand their scopes or practice. Provision of supplies can not only help to ensure access to clean supplies, but also help to develop a therapeutic relationship with patients.[73]

Other Preventative Measures: Vaccinations and Pre-exposure Prophylaxis for Human Immunodeficiency Virus Infection

Vaccinations
Hepatitis A, B, Td, and Tdap vaccines are indicated for PWID. Viral hepatitis vaccines may be given without serologic confirmation. PCV13 and PPSV23 vaccines should

also be offered to PWID who report tobacco or alcohol use. Other age-appropriate vaccines should be given per national guidelines.[74,75]

Pre-exposure prophylaxis
PWID are at risk for acquiring HIV infection; however, PrEP uptake for PWID has been relatively low.[76] Oral tenofovir disoproxil fumarate/emtricitabine and oral tenofovir alafenamide fumarate/emtricitabine taken once daily are both approved by the US Food and Drug Administration for PrEP, although oral tenofovir alafenamide fumarate/emtricitabine has not been studied in people at risk for HIV through receptive vaginal sex and there are cost concerns.[77] Although not yet approved by the US Food and Drug Administration, long-acting injectable formulations of PrEP may be future options.[78]

In addition to increasing provider knowledge and training around PrEP prescribing,[79] strategies such as developing electronic medical record-based algorithms to alert providers of potential PrEP candidates, colocating PrEP and other services, and creating pharmacist-led PrEP programs through collaborative practice agreements are feasible and acceptable approaches to integrating PrEP prescribing into clinical practice.[80–82]

Low barrier programs
Low barrier programs incorporate a harm reduction approach of meeting patients with SUD "where they are at." They can increase engagement in care, as well as improve patient–provider relationships and patient outcomes. These programs are flexible and meet the needs of individual patients, for example, maintaining SUD program participation even in the setting of continued drug use.[83] Although they may offer counseling services, low barrier programs do not require counseling. This harm reduction, patient-centered approach could also minimize infectious complications of IDU.[84] A lack of confidence has been cited as a provider barrier to providers offering SUD treatment[85]; however, there are several resources such as warmlines[86] and telemedicine programs for provider-to-provider consultation to help providers integrate SUD treatment into their practices.[87]

Prescribing heroin or fentanyl
In the United States, heroin cannot be prescribed. However, in other countries, prescribing heroin (also known as "supervised injectable heroin" or "heroin-assisted treatment") with optional oral methadone had benefits for people "refractory" to MOUD. Because the heroin is quality controlled (ie, of a known potency) and dosed at intervals based on patient response, this approach has been adopted to minimize overdose risk and engage PWID in care.[88]

In Canada, in PWID who are also refractory to MOUD, there is also some evidence on treating OUD with prescribed transdermal fentanyl, which creates stable, long-acting drug levels.[89] Although diversion and safety are valid concerns, transdermal fentanyl could prove to be another harm reduction approach to mitigate the downstream infectious complications of injecting fentanyl.[89]

Advocacy and partnering with the community
Medicaid expansion has been associated with increased naloxone availability and improved health outcomes.[90,91] In addition, Good Samaritan laws can protect people from prosecution if they help to reverse an overdose.[92] Providers can play an important role in advocating for Medicaid expansion and Good Samaritan laws in states where these policies have not yet been adopted. In addition, partnering with the community is key to help promoting best practices around harm reduction.[93,94] Finally,

especially in areas where harm reduction services are scarce or prohibited, providers can partner with community organizations to advocate for SSPs, SIFs, and other policies like eliminating 1-for-1syringe exchange and decriminalization of drug paraphernalia and syringe possession.

Summary

- Naloxone prescribing can be integrated into clinical practice
- Discussing safe injection techniques, offering vaccinations, and PrEP for HIV prevention are some evidence based-strategies for preventing IDU-associated infections
- Low barrier programs can improve engagement in care and patient outcomes
- Advocacy is crucial for promoting harm reduction

DISCUSSION

Harm reduction is grounded in social justice and aimed at meeting people where they are at. By integrating a harm reduction approach into practice, providers can help to mitigate the infectious complications of drug use. In addition to interacting with patients in a nonjudgmental manner and with compassion, providers should work with patients to develop practical strategies to minimize infectious consequences associated with drug use. By openly discussing safe injection techniques and access to harm reduction services such as SSPs, naloxone, and other drug equipment, providers can empower PWID to use more safely. Moreover, advocating for policies that increase access to harm reduction services, such as SIFs and elimination of 1-for-1 syringe exchanges, can help to ensure that PWID are able to access life-saving prevention and treatment services.

DISCLOSURE

The authors have no financial disclosures or conflicts of interest to report.

REFERENCES

1. Coalition HR. Principles of harm reduction. Available at: https://harmreduction. org/about-us/principles-of-harm-reduction/. Accessed March 10, 2020.
2. National Alliance of State and Territorial AIDS directors, Urban Coalition for HIV/ AIDS Prevention Services. Syringe services program (SSP) development and implementation guidelines for state and local health departments. 2012.
3. Chu Z, Xu J, Reilly KH, et al. HIV related high risk behaviors and willingness to participate in HIV vaccine trials among China MSM by computer assisted self-interviewing survey. Biomed Res Int 2013;2013:493128.
4. Gay Man's Health Crisis. Syringe exchange programs around the world: the global context. 2009. Available at: https://www.gmhc.org/files/editor/file/gmhc_ intl_seps.pdf. Accessed June 2020.
5. Guardino V, Des Jarlais, Arasteh K, et al. Syringe exchange programs — United States, 2008. MMWR Morb Mortal Wkly Rep 2010;59(45):1488–91.
6. Des Jarlais DC, McKnight C, Goldblatt C, et al. Doing harm reduction better: syringe exchange in the United States. Addiction 2009;104(9):1441–6.
7. Summers PJ, Hellman JL, MacLean MR, et al. Negative experiences of pain and withdrawal create barriers to abscess care for people who inject heroin. A mixed methods analysis. Drug Alcohol Depend 2018;190:200–8.

8. Tookes H, Bartholomew TS, Geary S, et al. Rapid Identification and Investigation of an HIV Risk Network Among People Who Inject Drugs -Miami, FL, 2018. AIDS Behav 2020;24(1):246–56.

9. Behrends CN, Nugent AV, Des Jarlais DC, et al. Availability of HIV and HCV On-Site Testing and Treatment at Syringe Service Programs in the United States. J Acquir Immun Defic Syndr 2018;79(2):e76–8.

10. Weinmeyer R. Needle Exchange Programs' Status in US Politics. AMA J Ethics 2016;18(3):252–7.

11. Burris S. Syringe Distribution Laws. Available at: http://lawatlas.org/datasets/syringe-policies-laws-regulating-non-retail-distribution-of-drug-parapherna. Accessed February 14, 2020.

12. Teshale EH, Asher A, Aslam MV, et al. Estimated cost of comprehensive syringe service program in the United States. PLoS One 2019;14(4):e0216205.

13. Des Jarlais DC, Nugent A, Solberg A, et al. Syringe Service Programs for Persons Who Inject Drugs in Urban, Suburban, and Rural Areas - United States, 2013. MMWR Morb Mortal Wkly Rep 2015;64(48):1337–41.

14. Phillips KT, Altman JK, Corsi KF, et al. Development of a risk reduction intervention to reduce bacterial and viral infections for injection drug users. Subst Use Misuse 2013;48(1–2):54–64.

15. MacArthur GJ, van Velzen E, Palmateer N, et al. Interventions to prevent HIV and Hepatitis C in people who inject drugs: a review of reviews to assess evidence of effectiveness. Int J Drug Policy 2014;25(1):34–52.

16. Fernandes RM, Cary M, Duarte G, et al. Effectiveness of needle and syringe Programmes in people who inject drugs - An overview of systematic reviews. BMC Public Health 2017;17(1):309.

17. Ruiz MS, O'Rourke A, Allen ST, et al. Using Interrupted Time Series Analysis to Measure the Impact of Legalized Syringe Exchange on HIV Diagnoses in Baltimore and Philadelphia. J Acquir Immun Defic Syndr 2019;82(Suppl 2):S148–54.

18. Allen ST, O'Rourke A, White RH, et al. Barriers and facilitators to PrEP use among people who inject drugs in rural Appalachia: a qualitative study. AIDS Behav 2019;24(6):1942–50.

19. Doerrbecker J, Behrendt P, Mateu-Gelabert P, et al. Transmission of hepatitis C virus among people who inject drugs: viral stability and association with drug preparation equipment. J Infect Dis 2013;207(2):281–7.

20. Palmateer NE, Taylor A, Goldberg DJ, et al. Rapid decline in HCV incidence among people who inject drugs associated with national scale-up in coverage of a combination of harm reduction interventions. PLoS One 2014;9(8):e104515.

21. Canary L, Hariri S, Campbell C, et al. Geographic Disparities in Access to Syringe Services Programs Among Young Persons With Hepatitis C Virus Infection in the United States. Clin Infect Dis 2017;65(3):514–7.

22. Platt L, Minozzi S, Reed J, et al. Needle and syringe programmes and opioid substitution therapy for preventing HCV transmission among people who inject drugs: findings from a Cochrane Review and meta-analysis. Addiction 2018;113(3):545–63.

23. Hagan H, Jarlais DC, Friedman SR, et al. Reduced risk of hepatitis B and hepatitis C among injection drug users in the Tacoma syringe exchange program. Am J Public Health 1995;85(11):1531–7.

24. Des Jarlais DC. Harm reduction in the USA: the research perspective and an archive to David Purchase. Harm Reduct J 2017;14(1):51.

25. SEP locations. 2020. Available at: https://www.nasen.org/map/. Accessed March 9, 2020.

26. Davis CS, Carr DH, Samuels EA. Paraphernalia Laws, Criminalizing Possession and Distribution of Items Used to Consume Illicit Drugs, and Injection-Related Harm. Am J Public Health 2019;109(11):1564–7.

27. Beletsky L, Davis CS, Anderson E, et al. The law (and politics) of safe injection facilities in the United States. Am J Public Health 2008;98(2):231–7.

28. Abuse CCoS. Needle exchange programs (NEPs) FAQs 2004.

29. Dolan K, Kimber J, Fry C, et al. Drug consumption facilities in Europe and the establishment of supervised injecting centres in Australia. Drug Alcohol Rev 2000;19(3):337–46.

30. Mema SC, Frosst G, Bridgeman J, et al. Mobile supervised consumption services in Rural British Columbia: lessons learned. Harm Reduct J 2019;16(1):4.

31. Mertz E, Bartko K. Edmonton supervised consumption site opening at Royal Alexandra Hospital April 2. 2018. Available at: https://globalnews.ca/news/4107666/royal-alexandra-hospital-safe-injection-supervised-consumption-site/. Accessed March 10, 2020.

32. Hyshka E, Strathdee S, Wood E, et al. Needle exchange and the HIV epidemic in Vancouver: lessons learned from 15 years of research. Int J Drug Policy 2012;23(4):261–70.

33. Hedrich D, Kerr T, Dubois-A. Drug Consumption Facilities in Europe and Beyond Harm Reduction: Evidence, Impacts and Challenges: European Monitoring Centre for Drugs and Drug Addiction. 2010. Available at: https://www.emcdda.europa.eu/system/files/publications/555/EMCDDA-monograph10-harm_reduction_final_205049.pdf. Accessed June 2020.

34. Marshall BD, Milloy MJ, Wood E, et al. Reduction in overdose mortality after the opening of North America's first medically supervised safer injecting facility: a retrospective population-based study. Lancet 2011;377(9775):1429–37.

35. Milloy MJ, Kerr T, Tyndall M, et al. Estimated drug overdose deaths averted by North America's first medically-supervised safer injection facility. PLoS One 2008;3(10):e3351.

36. Salmon AM, van Beek I, Amin J, et al. The impact of a supervised injecting facility on ambulance call-outs in Sydney, Australia. Addiction 2010;105(4):676–83.

37. Kilmer B, Taylor J, Caulkins JP, et al. Considering heroin-assisted treatment and supervised drug consumption sites in the United States. Santa Monica, CA:: RAND; 2018.

38. Kerr T, Tyndall MW, Lai C, et al. Drug-related overdoses within a medically supervised safer injection facility. Int J Drug Policy 2006;17(5):436–41.

39. Darke S, Ross J, Hall W. Overdose among heroin users in Sydney, Australia: I. Prevalence and correlates of non-fatal overdose. Addiction 1996;91(3):405–11.

40. Belackova V, Ritter A, Shanahan M, et al. Assessing the concordance between illicit drug laws on the books and drug law enforcement: comparison of three states on the continuum from "decriminalised" to "punitive". Int J Drug Policy 2017;41:148–57.

41. Lloyd-Smith E, Wood E, Zhang R, et al. Determinants of hospitalization for a cutaneous injection-related infection among injection drug users: a cohort study. BMC Public Health 2010;10:327.

42. Palepu A, Tyndall MW, Leon H, et al. Hospital utilization and costs in a cohort of injection drug users. CMAJ 2001;165(4):415–20.

43. Bayoumi AM, Zaric GS. The cost-effectiveness of Vancouver's supervised injection facility. CMAJ 2008;179(11):1143–51.

44. Pinkerton SD. How many HIV infections are prevented by Vancouver Canada's supervised injection facility? Int J Drug Policy 2011;22(3):179–83.

45. Andresen MA, Boyd N. A cost-benefit and cost-effectiveness analysis of Vancouver's supervised injection facility. Int J Drug Policy 2010;21(1):70–6.

46. Kerr T, Tyndall M, Li K, et al. Safer injection facility use and syringe sharing in injection drug users. Lancet 2005;366(9482):316–8.

47. Kennedy MC, Karamouzian M, Kerr T. Public health and public order outcomes associated with supervised drug consumption facilities: a systematic review. Curr HIV/AIDS Rep 2017;14(5):161–83.

48. Irwin A, Jozaghi E, Bluthenthal RN, et al. A cost-benefit analysis of a potential supervised injection facility in San Francisco, California, USA. J Drug Issues 2017;47(2):164–84.

49. Wood E, Tyndall MW, Qui Z, et al. Service uptake and characteristics of injection drug users utilizing North America's first medically supervised safer injecting facility. Am J Public Health 2006;96(5):770–3.

50. Stoltz J-A, Wood E, Small W, et al. Changes in injecting practices associated with the use of a medically supervised safer injection facility. J Public Health 2007;29(1):35–9.

51. Broadhead RS, Kerr TH, Grund J-PC, et al. Safer injection facilities in North America: their place in public policy and health initiatives. J Drug Issues 2002;32(1):329–55.

52. Wood E, Tyndall MW, Lai C, et al. Impact of a medically supervised safer injecting facility on drug dealing and other drug-related crime. Substance Abuse Treat Prev Policy 2006;1:13.

53. Kerr T, Stoltz JA, Tyndall M, et al. Impact of a medically supervised safer injection facility on community drug use patterns: a before and after study. BMJ 2006;332(7535):220–2.

54. Feldman N, Blumgart J. Safehouse hits pause on plan to open supervised injection site in South Phill. 2020. Available at: https://whyy.org/articles/safehouse-hits-pause-on-plan-to-open-supervised-injection-site-in-south-philly/. Accessed March 4, 2020.

55. Coffin PO, Sullivan SD. Cost-effectiveness of distributing naloxone to heroin users for lay overdose reversal in Russian cities. J Med Econ 2013;16(8):1051–60.

56. Walley AY, Xuan Z, Hackman HH, et al. Opioid overdose rates and implementation of overdose education and nasal naloxone distribution in Massachusetts: interrupted time series analysis. BMJ 2013;346:f174.

57. Prescribing Naloxone And Pharmacy Access To Naloxone In MA. Available at: http://masstapp.edc.org/prescribing-naloxone-and-pharmacy-access-naloxone-ma. Accessed March 10, 2020.

58. Lim JK, Bratberg JP, Davis CS, et al. Prescribe to prevent: overdose prevention and naloxone rescue kits for prescribers and pharmacists. J Addict Med 2016;10(5):300–8.

59. Drainoni ML, Koppelman EA, Feldman JA, et al. Why is it so hard to implement change? A qualitative examination of barriers and facilitators to distribution of naloxone for overdose prevention in a safety net environment. BMC Res Notes 2016;9(1):465.

60. Coffin PO, Behar E, Rowe C, et al. Nonrandomized intervention study of naloxone coprescription for primary care patients receiving long-term opioid therapy for pain. Ann Intern Med 2016;165(4):245–52.

61. Kispert D, Carwile JL, Silvia KB, et al. Differences in Naloxone Prescribing by Patient Age, Ethnicity, and Clinic Location Among Patients at High-Risk of Opioid Overdose. J Gen Intern Med 2020;35(5):1603–5.

62. Mueller SR, Walley AY, Calcaterra SL, et al. A review of opioid overdose prevention and naloxone prescribing: implications for translating community programming into clinical practice. Subs Abus 2015;36(2):240–53.

63. Albert S, Brason FW 2nd, Sanford CK, et al. Project Lazarus: community-based overdose prevention in rural North Carolina. Pain Med 2011;12(Suppl 2): S77–85.

64. Beletsky L, Ruthazer R, Macalino GE, et al. Physicians' knowledge of and willingness to prescribe naloxone to reverse accidental opiate overdose: challenges and opportunities. J Urban Health 2007;84(1):126–36.

65. Jawa R, Luu T, Bachman M, et al. Rapid naloxone administration workshop for health care providers at an academic medical center. MedEdPORTAL 2020;16: 10892.

66. Substance Abuse and Mental Health Services Administration. SAMHSA Opioid Overdose Prevention Toolkit. HHS Publication No. (SMA) 18–4742. Rockville, MD: Substance Abuse and Mental Health Services Administration, 2018.

67. Harm Reduction Coalition. Fentanyl test strip pilot: San Francisco (CA): 2018. Available at: https://harmreduction.org/issue-area/overdose-prevention-issue-area/fentanyl-test-strip-pilot/. Accessed March 2, 2020.

68. Peiper NC, Clarke SD, Vincent LB, et al. Fentanyl test strips as an opioid overdose prevention strategy: findings from a syringe services program in the Southeastern United States. Int J Drug Policy 2019;63:122–8.

69. Thakarar K, Weinstein ZM, Walley AY. Optimising health and safety of people who inject drugs during transition from acute to outpatient care: narrative review with clinical checklist. Postgrad Med J 2016;92(1088):356–63.

70. Seval N, Eaton E, Springer SA. Beyond antibiotics: a practical guide for the infectious disease physician to treat opioid use disorder in the setting of associated infectious diseases. Open Forum Infect Dis 2020;7(1):ofz539.

71. Phillips KT, Anderson BJ, Herman DS, et al. Risk factors associated with skin and soft tissue infections among hospitalized people who inject drugs. J Addict Med 2017;11(6):461–7.

72. Rhodes T. Risk environments and drug harms: a social science for harm reduction approach. Int J Drug Policy 2009;20(3):193–201.

73. Keyes KM, Cerda M, Brady JE, et al. Understanding the rural-urban differences in nonmedical prescription opioid use and abuse in the United States. Am J Public Health 2014;104(2):e52–9.

74. Belani H, Chorba T, Fletcher F, et al. Centers for Disease Control and Prevention. Integrated prevention services for HIV infection, viral hepatitis, sexually transmitted diseases, and tuberculosis for persons who use drugs illicitly: summary guidance from CDC and the U.S. Department of Health and Human Services. MMWR Recomm Rep 2012;61(RR-5):1–40.

75. Rockwell PG. ACIP Approves 2020 Adult and Childhood/Adolescent Immunization Schedules. Am Fam Physician 2020;101(4):251–2.

76. Taylor JL, Walley AY, Bazzi AR. Stuck in the window with you: HIV exposure prophylaxis in the highest risk people who inject drugs. Subs Abus 2019;40(4): 441–3.

77. Krakower DS, Daskalakis DC, Feinberg J, et al. Tenofovir alafenamide for HIV preexposure prophylaxis: what can we DISCOVER about its true value? Ann Intern Med 2020;172:281–2.

78. Marshall BDL, Goedel WC, King MRF, et al. Potential effectiveness of long-acting injectable pre-exposure prophylaxis for HIV prevention in men who have sex with men: a modelling study. Lancet HIV 2018;5(9):e498–505.

79. Christian ECW, Thakarar K. Examining PrEP knowledge and prescribing likelihood among medical residents before and after PrEP education. Open Forum Infect Dis 2018;5(suppl_1):S403.

80. Krakower DS, Gruber S, Hsu K, et al. Development and validation of an automated HIV prediction algorithm to identify candidates for pre-exposure prophylaxis: a modelling study. Lancet HIV 2019;6(10):e696–704.

81. Havens JP, Scarsi KK, Sayles H, et al. Acceptability and feasibility of a pharmacist-led HIV pre-exposure prophylaxis (PrEP) program in the Midwestern United States. Open Forum Infect Dis 2019;6(10).

82. Uyei J, Fiellin DA, Buchelli M, et al. Effects of naloxone distribution alone or in combination with addiction treatment with or without pre-exposure prophylaxis for HIV prevention in people who inject drugs: a cost-effectiveness modelling study. Lancet Public Health 2017;2(3):e133–40.

83. Martin SA, Chiodo LM, Bosse JD, et al. The next stage of buprenorphine care for opioid use disorder. Ann Intern Med 2019;170(11):821–2.

84. National Academies of Sciences E, and Medicine. Opportunities to improve opioid use disorder and infectious disease services: integrating responses to a dual epidemic. Washington, DC: The National Academies Press; 2020.

85. Andrilla CHA, Coulthard C, Patterson DG. Prescribing practices of rural physicians waivered to prescribe buprenorphine. Am J Prev Med 2018;54(6 Suppl 3):S208–14.

86. Egan JE, Casadonte P, Gartenmann T, et al. The Physician Clinical Support System-Buprenorphine (PCSS-B): a novel project to expand/improve buprenorphine treatment. J Gen Intern Med 2010;25(9):936–41.

87. Talal AH, Andrews P, McLeod A, et al. Integrated, co-located, telemedicine-based treatment approaches for hepatitis C virus management in opioid use disorder patients on methadone. Clin Infect Dis 2019;69(2):323–31.

88. Kilmer B, Taylor J, Caulkins JP, et al. Considering heroin-assisted treatment and supervised drug consumption sites in the United States. Santa Monica, CA: RAND Corporation; 2018.

89. Bardwell G, Wood E, Brar R. Fentanyl assisted treatment: a possible role in the opioid overdose epidemic? Substance Abuse Treat Prev Policy 2019;14(1):50.

90. Sohn M, Talbert JC, Delcher C, et al. Association between state Medicaid expansion status and naloxone prescription dispensing. Health Serv Res 2020;55(2):239–48.

91. Kravitz-Wirtz N, Davis CS, Ponicki WR, et al. Association of Medicaid Expansion With Opioid Overdose Mortality in the United States. JAMA Netw Open 2020;3(1):e1919066.

92. Jakubowski A, Kunins HV, Huxley-Reicher Z, et al. Knowledge of the 911 Good Samaritan Law and 911-calling behavior of overdose witnesses. Subs Abus 2018;39(2):233–8.

93. Associated Press. MMC research leads to toolkit for naloxone education. Portland Press Herald; 2019. Available at: https://www.pressherald.com/2019/10/31/researchers-naxolone-underprescribed-to-high-risk-patients/. Accessed June 2020

94. Davis C, Chang S, Carr D, et al. Legal interventions to reduce overdose mortality: naloxone access and overdose good Samaritan laws 2014. Network for

Public Health Law. Available at: https://www.networkforphl.org/wp-content/uploads/2020/01/legal-interventions-to-reduce-overdose.pdf. Accessed June 2020.

95. Bradford D, Jawa R, Wright J. Safer shooting: a harm reduction curriculum for patient centered advocacy in the treatment of people who inject drugs. Paper presented at: AMERSA; Boston, November 7, 2019.

96. Scott J, Winfield A, Kennedy E, et al. Laboratory study of the effects of citric and ascorbic acids on injections prepared with brown heroin. Int J Drug Policy 2000; 11(6):417–22.

97. Ng H, Patel RP, Bruno R, et al. Filtration of crushed tablet suspensions has potential to reduce infection incidence in people who inject drugs. Drug Alcohol Rev 2015;34(1):67–73.

98. Cruz MF, Patra J, Fischer B, et al. Public opinion towards supervised injection facilities and heroin-assisted treatment in Ontario, Canada. Int J Drug Policy 2007;18(1):54–61.

99. Lloyd-Smith E, Wood E, Zhang R, et al. Risk factors for developing a cutaneous injection-related infection among injection drug users: a cohort study. BMC Public Health 2008;8:405.

100. Hood JE, Behrends CN, Irwin A, et al. The projected costs and benefits of a supervised injection facility in Seattle, WA, USA. Int J Drug Policy 2019;67:9–18.

101. Irwin A, Jozaghi E, Weir BW, et al. Mitigating the heroin crisis in Baltimore, MD, USA: a cost-benefit analysis of a hypothetical supervised injection facility. Harm Reduct J 2017;14(1):29.

102. Ciccarone D, Harris M. Fire in the vein: heroin acidity and its proximal effect on users' health. Int J Drug Policy 2015;26(11):1103–10.

103. Coalition HR. A Safety Manual For Injection Drug Users. 2015. Available at: https://harmreduction.org/wp-content/uploads/2011/12/getting-off-right.pdf. Accessed Mar 4, 2020.

104. Harris M, Scott J, Wright T, et al. Injecting-related health harms and overuse of acidifiers among people who inject heroin and crack cocaine in London: a mixed-methods study. Harm Reduct J 2019;16(1):60.

105. Harris M. The 'do-it-yourself' New Zealand injecting scene: implications for harm reduction. Int J Drug Policy 2013;24(4):281–3.

106. Coalition HR. Overdose Prevention Tips. Available at: https://harmreduction.org/wp-content/uploads/2012/11/HRC_ODprevention_worksheet9.pdf. Accessed March 2 2020.

Improving Outpatient Management of Patients On Chronic Opioid Therapy

Jonathan A. Colasanti, MD, MSPH[a],*, Theresa Vettese, MD[b],
Jeffrey H. Samet, MD, MA, MPH[c,d]

KEYWORDS

- Chronic opioid therapy (COT) • Outpatient opioid management • Safe prescribing

KEY POINTS

- Chronic opioid therapy may be appropriate as part of a comprehensive pain management plan for persons with chronic pain.
- The risk-benefit ratio should be discussed and weighed on an ongoing basis to determine a monitoring and safety plan.
- Managing chronic opioid therapy can be accomplished safely and in concordance with guidelines, through a team-based approach.
- A comprehensive monitoring plan includes a goal-oriented and safety-based treatment agreement.

BACKGROUND

The Opioid Epidemic

The impact of the opioid epidemic in the United States has been devastating to individuals and communities. Over the last 18 years, more than 700,000 people in the United States have died of a drug overdose—two-thirds involved an opioid. Death from opioid overdose is six times higher than it was in 1999 and about one-third of those are attributable to an overdose related specifically to prescription opioids.[1] Increasing opioid deaths over the last 20 years are a consequence of 3 major events in the recent opioid

[a] Department of Medicine, Division of Infectious Diseases, Emory University, 341 Ponce de Leon Avenue, Atlanta, GA 30308, USA; [b] Department of Medicine, Division of General Internal Medicine and Geriatrics, Emory University, 49 Jesse Hill Drive SE #40, Atlanta, GA 30303, USA; [c] Clinical Addiction Research and Education Unit, Section of General Internal Medicine, Department of Medicine, Boston University School of Medicine, Boston Medical Center; 801 Massachusetts Avenue, CT 2, Boston, MA 02118, USA; [d] Department of Community Health Sciences, Boston University School of Public Health, 801 Massachusetts Avenue, CT 2, Boston, MA 02118, USA
* Corresponding author.
E-mail address: jcolasa@emory.edu
Twitter: @jcolasantimd (J.A.C.); @tracyvettese (T.V.)

Infect Dis Clin N Am 34 (2020) 621–635
https://doi.org/10.1016/j.idc.2020.06.014
0891-5520/20/© 2020 Elsevier Inc. All rights reserved.

epidemic history: increased prescription opioids in the 1990s, increased heroin use starting in 2010 as prescription opioids became less accessible, and finally a surge of synthetic opioids in 2013.[2] Opioid prescribing peaked in 2012 with about 81.3 prescriptions per 100 persons, which has subsequently declined to 58.7 per 100 in 2017. Yet although national declines are observed, opioid prescriptions rates in some counties are 7 times the national average, indicating high-risk areas.[3] For example, those in rural areas are much more likely to receive an opioid prescription.[4]

Opioid prescription declines have coincided with the Centers for Disease Control and Prevention's (CDC) first release of a *Guidelines for Prescribing Opioids for Chronic Pain*.[5] Although it is clear that overprescribing of opioids has been a problem nationwide, the exact role prescribers play in the nation's opioid epidemic is still debated. Through education efforts, promulgation of the abovementioned CDC guidelines and the roll out of state prescription drug monitoring programs (PDMPs), opioid prescribing for chronic pain is less commonly pursued.[6] When opioid therapy is continued for longer than 90 days, as part of pain management, it is referred to as chronic opioid therapy (COT) or long-term opioid therapy. Stopping COT for pain does not come without risk, as discontinuation of therapy has been associated with overdose and transition to illicit opioids.[7] In response to such data plus anecdotes of suicide due to poorly controlled pain after forced opioid tapers, the CDC recently acknowledged potential harmful unintended consequences of the clinical practice changes that the guidelines may have precipitated.[8] Subsequently, the Department of Health and Human Services issued formal guidance on tapering and individualizing opioid therapy, discouraging forced tapers and emphasizing that it is ok to continue opioid therapy when benefits outweigh risks.[9]

Chronic Pain and Its Challenges

In the midst of an ongoing opioid epidemic and debates about how best to address opioid prescribing, the United States also suffers from an epidemic of chronic pain. Using National Health Interview Survey data, the CDC estimates that 20.4% (50 million) adults in the United States suffered from chronic pain in 2016 and almost 20 million adults reported high-impact chronic pain, defined as pain that limit life or work activities on most days during the prior 6 months.[10,11] Furthermore, disparities emerged with women, older adults, those living in poverty, those with less than high school degree, the unemployed (previously worked), the publicly insured, and rural residents being disproportionately affected.[10]

Opioids are not recommended as initial therapy for chronic pain nor do robust data support the efficacy of opioids for the management of chronic pain.[5,12,13] Yet, based on clinical experience and survey-based studies, some patients clearly report improvement in pain, function, and quality of life with opioid therapy.[14–16] Unfortunately, clinicians lack tools to a-priori identify for which patients the opioid therapy will or will not be effective. Clinicians are left using a stepwise approach to pain management, at times arriving at opioids and COT as a part of the ongoing pain management plan. Clinicians are faced with daily decisions concerning managing patients' pain in a less than supportive environment of regulators and systems seeking to curb opioid prescribing. Although physicians take an oath to *do no harm* we also have an obligation to address our patients' health concerns and at times that is principally pain. And yet our overarching health system is often not structured in a way that facilitates access to multidisciplinary pain management. The challenge of alleviating pain then rests with the primary care clinicians, often uncomfortably.

In general, primary care clinicians feel uncomfortable or ill equipped to manage chronic pain and specifically the management of COT. This discomfort stems largely from lack of training throughout their medical education careers and lack of support staff such as multidisciplinary teams.[17–19] Yet, given the reality of practice, it is often the primary care clinician who prescribes and manages COT for chronic pain. The infectious diseases (ID) workforce is disproportionately confronted with this dilemma in the setting of longitudinal management of persons with human immunodeficiency virus (HIV) where the ID clinician is often the primary care provider.[20] The Infectious Disease Society of American and the HIV Medical Association recognized this challenge for their workforce, responding with the publication of the *2017 HIVMA of IDSA Clinical Practice Guideline for the Management of Chronic Pain in Patients Living with HIV.*[21] This document, with respect to opioids, is largely in line with the broader CDC *Guidelines for Prescribing Opioids for Chronic Pain.* In persons with HIV, suboptimal pain management is associated with poor retention in care and virologic failure, suggesting the need for improved access to clinicians trained in and comfortable with managing chronic pain, including managing COT.[22] Given the importance of pain management in HIV care and that managing chronic pain in the primary care setting can be challenging for those with minimal formal related training (eg, addiction medicine, pain management, or palliative care), we aim for this piece to be a practical tool in the care of patients on COT.

In this article, the authors highlight important aspects of managing patients on COT and provide a roadmap for practicing clinicians and clinical staff managing patients with chronic pain on COT (**Table 1**).

APPROACH TO CHRONIC PAIN
Patient Assessment and Goal Setting

All patients presenting with chronic pain should have a thorough assessment including a detailed "pain" history, which includes inciting injury or event and what treatments have been tried alone or in combination as well as their effects and adverse consequences. A focused physical examination should be performed as well as appropriate imaging tests. It is ideal to identify a specific diagnosis for the patient's pain, as different causes respond differently to certain treatments. Because depression and anxiety are common comorbidities with chronic pain, all patients should be screened using a validated instrument and treated for both.

Following a thorough assessment for chronic pain, clinicians should assist patients in establishing functional and quality-of-life goals that can be used as the major measure of the effectiveness of the pain management program. Establishing baseline measures of pain and function allows longitudinal assessment and objective monitoring for improvement. Functional goals can include emotional dimensions (eg, interactions with family and friends, spiritual) or physical (eg, work, leisure, sexual, sleep) and should follow the SMART goal framework: Specific, Measurable, Achievable, Relevant, and Time-bound.[5,23,24] Although measurement of pain relief is important, clinicians should be clear in discussing these expectations with patients. Progress toward these patient-centered goals should be considered a positive response to treatment modalities including opioid pain medication (OPM). Some clinicians may opt to use a validated tool to measure treatment effectiveness, such as the 3-item Pain average, interference with Enjoyment of life, and interference with General activity (PEG) assessment scale, which is easy to use in the primary care setting.[25]

ALTERNATIVE PHARMACOLOGIC AGENTS AND MODALITIES OF TREATMENT

Nonpharmacologic and nonopioid therapy should be the preferred strategies for the treatment of chronic pain.[5] Multiple nonpharmacologic and nonopioid treatments

Table 1
Concise summary and resources for managing patients on chronic opioid therapy

Key Steps and Principles When Initiating Opioid/Chronic Opioid Therapy	Links to Related Resources
General resources for education and guidance around opioid prescribing.	Scope of Pain: safer/competent opioid prescribing education: https://www.scopeofpain.org myTopCare: guide for physicians and pharmacists in care for patients on chronic opioid therapy for chronic pain http://mytopcare.org
Basic Principles • Stepwise approach to chronic pain management with nonopioids first • Lowest effective dose, slow titration • Objective evaluation for improved function and quality of life • Frequent reassessment of risk/benefit profile	https://www.cdc.gov/drugoverdose/pdf/nonopioid_treatments-a.pdf PEG (*Pain* average, interference with *Enjoyment* of life, interference with *General* activity) http://mytopcare.org/wp-content/uploads/2013/06/PEG-Pain-Screening-Tool1.pdf
Treatment agreement • Informed decision that weighs risks/benefits and states intended use and benefit • Outlines patient expectations, monitoring strategy, and refill plan	http://mytopcare.org/prescribers/starting-opioids/creating-and-using-a-treatment-plan/
Risk Stratification Tools • Pain Medication Questionnaire (PMQ), 26 items • Opioid Risk Tool (ORT), 6 items • Screener and Opioid Assessment for Patients with Pain-Revised (SOAPP-R), 24 items • Current Opioid Misuse Measure (COMM), 17 items	PMQ: https://www.jpsmjournal.com/article/S0885-3924(04)00101-0/fulltext ORT: https://www.drugabuse.gov/sites/default/files/opioidrisktool.pdf SOAPP-R: https://www.helpisherede.com/Content/Documents/SOAPP-Tool.pdf COMM: http://mytopcare.org/wp-content/uploads/2013/05/COMM.pdf

Urine Drug Testing
• Key history for interpretation:
  ○ Substances (prescription and non) currently taking
  ○ Dose/interval and when was last dose in relation to UDT
• Assistance with interpretation based on prescribed opioid
• Understand how to interpret results in context of what is expected vs unexpected
	http://mytopcare.org/prescribers/about-urine-drug-tests/
	http://mytopcare.org/urine-drug-test-overview/

Naloxone Co-prescription • Consider for patients with history of: • Overdose or substance use disorder • Daily morphine milliequivalent ≥50 • Co-prescribed benzodiazepine	

(continued on next page)

Table 1 (continued)	
Key Steps and Principles When Initiating Opioid/Chronic Opioid Therapy	**Links to Related Resources**
DSM-V Criteria for Opioid Use Disorder in Setting of COT: **Mild (2–3), Moderate (4–5), Severe (≥6)**	
1. Opioids used in larger amounts or for longer than intended 2. Persistent desire or unsuccessful efforts to cut down on opioid use 3. Great deal of time spent trying to obtain, use or recover from the effects of the opioid 4. Craving	5. Failing to meet major obligations or responsibilities 6. Continued use despite persistent social or interpersonal problems related to the opioid use 7. Activities given up due to opioid use 8. Recurrent opioid use in hazardous situations 9. Persistent use despite ongoing physical or psychological problems as a result of the use
Taper Strategy (see **Box 1**)	https://www.cdc.gov/drugoverdose/pdf/clinical_pocket_guide_tapering-a.pdf https://www.hhs.gov/opioids/sites/default/files/2019-10/Dosage_Reduction_Discontinuation.pdf

have been shown to be modestly effective for various types of chronic pain. Cognitive behavioral therapy has been demonstrated to enhance mood and decrease catastrophizing in chronic nonheadache pain and also seems to be similarly effective whether it is internet delivered or face-to-face.[26,27] Exercise therapy demonstrates modest improvement in pain and physical function in various causes of chronic pain with few adverse effects.[28] Acetaminophen is more effective than placebo for management of osteoarthritis but not as effective as nonsteroidal antiinflammatory drugs (NSAIDs).[29] NSAIDs are also helpful for chronic lower back pain.[30–32] Although NSAIDs have been associated with gastrointestinal, renal, and cardiovascular complications, they are likely underutilized as analgesics. Multiple effective strategies exist to decrease gastrointestinal and cardiovascular risks of NSAIDs, and low-dose use has been demonstrated to be safe in most of the patients with chronic kidney disease.[33–36] Gabapentenoids can be helpful for the management of diabetic neuropathy and postherpetic neuralgia but have been increasingly prescribed for off-label indications and have significant adverse effects.[37] Interdisciplinary multimodality chronic pain management programs offer the best results for patients but unfortunately are not widely available despite demonstrating cost-effectiveness.[38]

HOW AND WHEN TO INITIATE OPIOIDS

In patients with functionally limiting chronic pain who have failed to respond to multiple nonopioid and nonpharmacologic therapies and in whom potential benefits are likely to outweigh risk, a trial of low-dose OPM can be considered. OPM should be used in combination with other nonpharmacologic and nonopioid pharmacologic treatments. When communicating with patients about OPM, clinicians should adopt a patient-centered risk versus benefit approach. In this approach the clinician judges the opioid treatment, not the patient.[39] Continuing the trial of OPM is based on whether it is beneficial, and risks are minimal. Changing the treatment plan is about keeping the patient safe.[40] The initial step should be to clearly discuss the potential risks and benefits of OPM. Data regarding the long-term benefit of COT in chronic pain are not convincing but individual patients may achieve modest improvement in function.[41]

Providing COT is best done in the context of a therapeutic relationship. The initial step should be to clearly discuss the potential risks and benefits of OPM. A risk-benefit discussion focuses on the opioid therapy itself carrying the risk rather than portraying patients themselves as carrying the risk. Risk-benefit discussions are best when clear and objective. The risks of OPM are significant and include unintentional overdose and death, addiction, diversion, sedation, fatigue, constipation, sexual dysfunction, osteoporosis, and immunosuppression.[5,42] Adverse effects include dry mouth, constipation, drowsiness, confusion, nausea, vomiting, and respiratory suppression. Tolerance and physical dependence are expected in the setting of chronic use of opioids. A dose-dependent risk of overdose exists and increases significantly at a dose of greater than 50 morphine milliequivalents (MME) as well as in the setting of concomitant benzodiazepine therapy.[43,44]

Before considering a trial of low-dose OPM, patients should be screened for the risk of developing aberrant behaviors when prescribed OPM. There is no single gold-standard screening instrument but common ones include the Opioid Risk Tool (ORT),[45] the Screener and Opioid Assessment for Patients with Pain (SOAPP),[46] The Pain Medication Questionnaire (PMQ),[47] or the Current Opioid Misuse Measure (COMM).[48] In a systematic review, SOAPP and PMQ had the best evidence for predicting prescription opioid misuse, whereas the COMM performed best at screening for current misuse.[49] The ORT has the advantage of brevity (6 items), compared with the other instruments that have between 17 and 24 questions.[49] The tools themselves attempt to predict and risk stratify who will go on to misuse or is currently misusing. Patients who score in the high-risk category should have physicians and other prescribers consider very carefully before turning to this last option (OPM). If OPM is prescribed risk mitigation strategies should be adopted (see below). Opioids should be prescribed at the lowest effective dosage, only immediate-release OPM should be prescribed and dosages above 50 mg MME should be avoided.

Once a clinical decision is made for ongoing opioid prescriptions as part of a pain management plan or if a patient is inherited on COT, it is important to clarify expectations of such therapy, establish understanding of potential risks and harms of opioid therapy and develop a standard monitoring plan. A comprehensive risk-benefit discussion sets the stage for entering into a treatment agreement and allows for a monitoring discussion largely framed around patient and public safety as opposed to "policing" or "penalizing" the patient. The treatment agreement serves as an informed consent document outlining potential benefit and all risks/safety issues of OPM.[5,21]

TREATMENT AGREEMENTS AND MONITORING

As part of the discussion around risks and benefits, it is essential that all parties involved recognize that the clinical team and the patient hold joint responsibility in monitoring and mitigating risks of therapy. It is helpful to firmly establish that responsibility through a formalized treatment plan and opioid treatment agreement, signed by a member of the clinical team and the patient. Key aspects of a treatment plan include the following: (1) documenting other aspects of care that may help address the patient's chronic pain such as exercise or cognitive behavioral therapy, (2) documenting potential risks of therapy and intended benefits, (3) adhering to follow-up appointments, (4) potential for pill counts, (5) urine drug testing (UDT), (6) PDMP, (7) single prescriber and pharmacy for opioid dispensing, and (8) expectations around refills. More guidance on an in-depth assessment as part of a treatment plan is available at (http://mytopcare.org/prescribers/starting-opioids/creating-and-using-a-treatment-plan/). It is not entirely clear whether a treatment agreement in and of itself mitigates opioid misuse[50] but it is recognized as a best practice in guidelines.[21] When done universally and empathically with patients, a signed agreement, including consent and treatment plan, provides a framework for the entire monitoring process without singling out particular individuals, based on risk.[51] Importantly, a violation of that agreement does not necessarily equate cessation or immediate tapering of COT; however, the agreement does provide a platform for discussion and reassessment of risk benefits, which in turn informs a decision on how to proceed with further therapy. Although ideal that this is all done from the outset of COT, clinicians inheriting a patient already on COT should reestablish goals of therapy and treatment agreements at that point in time.

FOLLOW-UP AND CONTINUITY OF CARE

Clinical follow-up and monitoring are a central tenet of any chronic pain/opioid treatment plan. CDC recommends that patients are reevaluated for benefits and harms of therapy within 4 weeks of initiating therapy or dose change and then on a quarterly basis when on stable therapy.[5] Clinical follow-up in this case encompasses reviewing and reassessing risks and benefits on a continuous basis with patients.

Although the CDC endorses monitoring of the state PDMP and UDTs, pill counts are also often used as a part of a monitoring plan. Guidelines do not formally address exactly how frequently and what mix of monitoring should be used and in what scenarios. The online clinical aid, myTopcare, provides evidence-based guidance to prescribers around monitoring activities, including a range of frequencies for monitoring, increasing the risk profile of the patient (**Table 2**). Choosing how often to perform each monitoring strategy can be guided by using aforementioned risk assessment tools to risk stratify patients. Other clinical conditions that carry increased risks and may warrant more frequent monitoring include pregnancy, sleep-disordered breathing, renal or hepatic insufficiency, age greater than or equal to 65 years, comorbid mental health condition, or substance use. Furthermore, the dose of opioids may inform frequency of monitoring, given the association of doses of greater than or equal to 50 MME, and especially close follow-up with MME doses of greater than or equal to 90.[5] Ultimately, the final plan for the extent and frequency of monitoring should be informed by using a

---

Table 2
myTopCare recommended risk monitoring schedule per year for urine drug tests, prescription drug monitoring program review, pill counts, and primary care visits

Risk Level	UDTs	PDMP	Pill Counts	Minimum Primary Care Visits
Low risk/first 12 mo of treatment	1–3	1–3	1	4
Low	1–2	1	0	4
Moderate	3–4	3	1–2	4
High	Min 6—up to every prescription	4	3+	6

Abbreviations: PDMP, prescription drug monitoring program; UDTs, urine drug tests.
Adapted from mytopcare.org; with permission.

validated risk prediction tool, clinical judgment, the PDMP, and any other available data (eg, UDTs).[52]

VISIT FREQUENCY AND PILL COUNTS

Under the Drug Enforcement Administration's "valid prescription requirement," schedule II substances cannot be refilled but patients are permitted to receive up to 90 days of prescription that can be filled before seeing the prescriber again. Therefore, the patient is expected to see the prescribing provider at least quarterly to receive ongoing opioid therapy. Although this adheres to federal regulations, jurisdiction or institutional requirements may differ. Increased frequency of visits should be considered for those with higher risk of overdose or opioid misuse.

Pill counts may be particularly useful in determining exact patient adherence, dose self-escalation, and as a way to monitor for diversion. Pill counts are best conducted in the presence of the patient with a clear understanding of the date the medication was filled, interval it was prescribed, number of pills dispensed, and number that should be remaining.

URINE DRUG TESTING

UDT is one of the most useful and at times challenging aspects of monitoring COT for both patients and clinicians. In order for clinicians to properly interpret a UDT, it is important to document the dose and schedule, time of last dose in relation to the urine collection, and the patient's report of any other substances that might be detected on the test. For patients, it can feel stigmatizing and also require extra time. Framing the urine assessment as part of the determination of risk benefit and the treatment agreement discussions in terms of patient safety allows the clinician to explain how UDTs help assess the patient's risk using COT. In addition, it is important to emphasize the universality of the monitoring practice for those on COT, as this standardization of clinical practice should mitigate the stigma of UDTs. For the clinician, the UDT is one of the few pieces of objective data we can collect to inform our assessments around risk. UDTs can inform the clinician as to whether a patient is appropriately taking a prescribed opioid as well as whether co-occurring (nonprescribed) substance use exists.

Although this review is not intended to provide a comprehensive overview of the pharmacokinetics/dynamics that affect UDT interpretation, it is important to keep in mind the basic metabolism pathways of commonly used drugs (**Fig. 1**). Codeine, heroin, morphine, and hydrocodone all share the common metabolite of hydromorphone and are typically detectable by common UDT immunoassays (detection of opiates at

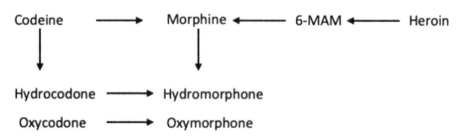

Fig. 1. Metabolic pathway of select semisynthetic and synthetic opioids. 6MAM, 6 monoacetylmorphine. (*Adapted from* mytopcare.org; with permission.)

concentrations of 300 ng/dL). Oxycodone has a distinct metabolic pathway such that common UDT opiate immunoassay screens will not detect it; a specific assay to detect oxymorphone is also needed. More detailed information on interpreting UDTs in the context of a variety of chronic opioid prescriptions can be found at mytopcare.com (http://mytopcare.org/udt-calculator/suspected-opioid-misuse/)

PRESCRIPTION DRUG MONITORING PROGRAM

The CDC guidelines make a specific recommendation to review the PDMP at least every 3 months. The PDMPs are state level databases that track controlled substance prescriptions. This facilitates monitoring of who is writing prescriptions for what, where they are filled, and who is filling them. At a clinician level it allows one to review whether your patient is receiving controlled substances from other prescribers in the state and many state databases now link together so one can monitor prescriptions from other states also. In some instances, the PDMP access is integrated in the electronic health record to improve efficiencies by minimizing clicks or sign-ins to separate websites for the treatment team. Each state has their own regulations around the governing and access of the PDMP, and prescribers/care teams should be familiar with their specific programs and jurisdictional level regulations of when and how frequently the database is required to be reviewed. The PDMP training and technical assistance center provides resources and links to each specific state program (https://www.pdmpassist. org/content/state-profiles). The impact of use of PDMPs on individual level prescribing behavior is mixed.[53]

TAKING ACTION
Overdose Prevention

Overdose prevention should be considered a dimension of the effort to decrease the risk of prescribing COT. Opioid overdose prevention begins with educating patients about this inherent risk of the development of tolerance to the analgesic property of opioid therapy and yet the ongoing risk of the pharmacologic suppression of respiratory drive. An accompanying naloxone prescription should be considered for patients at elevated risk of overdose such as history of an overdose, history of substance use disorder, high-dose opioid therapy ($\geq$50 MME), or coprescription of a benzodiazepine.

Another key aspect of the safety discussion with patients on COT should include keeping the medications out of reach of children or others in the home, and this can be achieved by keeping medications in a locked-cabinet and pursuing proper disposal of unused medication. Naloxone prescription should also accompany a prescription for someone who may be at low risk for overdose themselves but has a scenario where accidental overdose is possible from someone other than the patient getting into the medications.

Addiction Monitoring and Treatment

Part of comprehensive monitoring includes screening for addiction, referral for effective therapy, or provision of medications when SUD is diagnosed. The DSM-V criteria for opioid use disorder in the presence of COT requires 2 of the following criteria: (1) opioids used in larger amounts or for longer than intended, (2) persistent desire or unsuccessful efforts to cut down on opioid use, (3) great deal of time spent trying to obtain, use, or recover from the effects of the opioid, (4) craving, (5) failing to meet major obligations or responsibilities, (6) continued use despite persistent social or interpersonal problems related to the opioid use, (7) activities given up due to opioid use, (8) recurrent opioid use in hazardous situations, and (9) persistent use despite ongoing physical or psychological problems as the result of the use. The disorder is classified into mild (2–3 criteria), moderate (4–5 criteria), or severe (≥6 criteria).[54] These criteria exclude tolerance and withdrawal because those are physiologic and expected in setting of COT prescribed for analgesia. For patients exhibiting signs of opioid use disorder, referral to an addiction subspecialty physician and/or prescription of medications for opioid use disorder (ie, methadone, buprenorphine, or injectable naltrexone) should be considered.

DECREASING DOSES AND TAPERS

One tenet of optimizing COT is using the lowest effective dose. The Veteran Health Administration implemented an opioid safety initiative in 2013 using a dashboard to track metrics with the aim to decrease the number of patients receiving high-dose opioids (≥100 MME) and those receiving a concurrent benzodiazepine.[55] Each clinical site had a key leader responsible for reviewing reports and providing directed feedback to prescribers with clinical appropriateness determined on a case-by-case basis. Although initiatives to decrease opioid prescribing in general and especially in higher risk cases are important, we must ensure that those who warrant ongoing opioid therapy are managed in a nonstigmatizing, unbiased way with optimized safety and adherence monitoring. When the risks of OPM outweigh any potential benefit for an individual patient, OPM should be tapered: when a patient experiences intolerable side effects of OPM, failure to meet functional and quality-of-life goals for treatment, evidence of misuse, or resolution of pain. Again, the clinician should emphasize that tapering is due to the increased risk-to-benefit ratio of the OPM and is not intended as a judgment of the patient. A systematic review found low-quality evidence suggesting that several types of opioid tapers may result in decreased pain and increased function and better quality of life, which was especially true when provided via a multidisciplinary care team and with close follow-up.[56] All studies included only patients who voluntarily consented to taper.[56] The investigators do not advise tapering OPM in patients on long-term opioid therapy for chronic pain who have functional improvement and in whom risks are minimal. There are several guides to providing safe and comfortable opioid tapering for patients.[56,57] One such effective strategy is to decrease 10% of the original OPM dose every 5 to 7 days until 30% of the total original dose is reached, followed by a weekly decrease by 10% of the remaining dose.[57] The authors provide a case example in **Box 1**. Although precipitated withdrawal was rarely seen with this protocol, nonopioid strategies for withdrawal management may help with mild symptoms. Tapering speed should correlate with the duration of long-term opioid therapy and for some patients, dosage adjustments may need to be bimonthly or monthly. Consideration should be given to slowing the taper during times of stress or if withdrawal symptoms are problematic.

TEAM-BASED APPROACH AND MULTICOMPONENT INTERVENTIONS

Guideline concordant monitoring can be accomplished through a multicomponent intervention that includes education, team-based care, and systems-level changes. Two randomized controlled trials, one in the context of general primary care (TOPCARE) and one in the context of HIV primary care (TEACH), demonstrated comanagement and monitoring of the COT improved clinician adherence to guideline-recommended monitoring therapy. Specifically, components of this care included a nurse care manager, an electronic registry to guide nurse care manager monitoring activities, academic detailing for clinicians, and access to a pain/addiction specialist to discuss challenging cases.[58] The multicomponent intervention in primary care improved guidelines concordant care overall (adjusted odds ratio

---

Box 1
Example of 12-week tapering schedule for patient managed with chronic opioid therapy

Patient taking long-term opioid therapy for chronic pain:
- Oxycodone sustained-release (SR) 30 mg orally q 12 hours = 60 mg
- Oxycodone immediate-release (IR) 10 mg orally q 6 hours = 40 mg
- Total daily oxycodone dose = 100 mg

Week 1: reduce by 10% of the original daily dose (10 mg) = 100 mg − 10 mg = 90 mg
- Continue oxycodone SR 30 mg orally q 12 hours
- Oxycodone IR 10 mg q 8 hours

Week 2 to 4: repeat weekly dose decrease by 10% of original total dose (10 mg)

Week 4: total daily dose = 60 mg = convert oxycodone SR 30 mg q 12 hours to oxycodone IR 10 mg q 4 hours

Week 4–6: taper dose weekly by 10% of total original dose until 30% of original total dose is reached (30 mg)
- Convert oxycodone SR 30 mg orally q 12 hours to oxycodone IR 10 mg orally q 4 hours
- Decrease to oxycodone IR 10 mg orally q 5 hours for 5 total daily doses, then 10 mg orally q6 hours for 4 total daily doses, then 10 mg orally q8 hours for 3 total daily doses

Week 6: total daily dose = 30 mg = convert oxycodone IR 10 mg q 8 hours to oxycodone IR 5 mg orally q 4 hours

Week 6 to 12: taper dose weekly by 10% of remaining dose (approximately 5 mg) until off
- Convert oxycodone IR 10 mg orally q hours to oxycodone IR 5 mg orally q 4 hours
- Decrease to oxycodone IR 5 mg orally q 5 hours for 5 total daily doses, the 5 mg orally q6 hours for 4 total daily doses, then 5 mg orally q8 hours for 3 total daily doses, then 5 mg orally q12 hours for 2 total daily doses, then 5 mg orally daily for single daily dose

Other Tips
- Taper duration should be adjusted for duration of long-term therapy, for example, bimonthly or monthly dose decreases for long durations
- Taper should be slowed during times of patient stress or withdrawal symptoms
- Nonopioid pharmacologic strategies (eg, alpha blockers) should be used as adjuvant treatment of withdrawal symptoms

Abbreviations: IR, immediate-release; SR, sustained-release.

[AOR] 6.0; 95% confidence interval [CI], 3.6–10.2) and specifically increased patients with a pain agreement (AOR 11.9; 95% CI 4.4–32.2) and recommended UDTs (AOR 3.0; 95% CI, 1.8–5.0). In addition, patients who received the intervention were more likely than the control group to have 10% reduction in dose of opioids or treatment discontinuation (AOR 1.6; 95% CI, 1.3–2.1).[59] In a similar trial in HIV primary care settings, the multicomponent intervention had higher odds of having a pain agreement (AOR 128.11; 95%CI, 22.85–719.30) and receiving more than or equal to 2 UDTs (AOR 15.46; CI, 7.29–32.79).[60] Importantly, enhanced monitoring did not affect HIV viral suppression as is sometimes feared by HIV clinicians.[61] Furthermore, HIV clinicians receiving the nurse care manager support, academic detailing, and access to pain/addiction specialist had higher satisfaction and confidence scores around prescribing COT, whereas patients did not experience decreased satisfaction with care nor decreased trust in providers.[62]

SUMMARY

Summing up the CDC guidelines on paper can be succinctly stated: opioids are not the first-line treatment of pain management but when they are used, risks and benefits should be reviewed frequently with the patient. Use opioids in the lowest effective dose for shortest amount of time necessary. Opioids should be used in conjunction with risk mitigation practices and monitoring where overdose prevention is available, and addiction is treated with evidence-based approaches, when uncovered. Operationalizing optimal opioid management can be more challenging in routine clinical practice, especially in understaffed and underresourced settings. Multicomponent interventions[58–60,62] provide enhanced levels of education to clinicians prescribing opioid therapy, active nursing support to assist with risk assessment and monitoring, and access to experts to discuss challenging cases. These interventions can improve monitoring without severing clinician-patient trust and relationships.

DISCLOSURE

(J.A.C) This work was supported by the Center for AIDS Research at Emory University, P30AI050409; (J.A.C and J.H.S) this work was supported by National Institute of Drug Abuse (NIDA) 1R01DA037768-01.

REFERENCES

1. Scholl L, Seth P, Kariisa M, et al. Drug and opioid-involved overdose deaths - United States, 2013-2017. MMWR Morb Mortal Wkly Rep 2018;67(5152): 1419–27.
2. Kolodny A, Courtwright DT, Hwang CS, et al. The prescription opioid and heroin crisis: a public health approach to an epidemic of addiction. Annu Rev Public Health 2015;36:559–74.
3. CDC. U.S. Opioid Prescribing Rate Maps. Available at: https://www.cdc.gov/drugoverdose/maps/rxrate-maps.html. Accessed January 16, 2020.
4. Garcia MC, Heilig CM, Lee SH, et al. Opioid prescribing rates in nonmetropolitan and metropolitan counties among primary care providers using an electronic health record system - United States, 2014-2017. MMWR Morb Mortal Wkly Rep 2019;68(2):25–30.
5. Dowell D, Haegerich TM, Chou R. CDC guideline for prescribing opioids for chronic pain - United States, 2016. MMWR Recomm Rep 2016;65(1):1–49.
6. Bohnert ASB, Guy GP Jr, Losby JL. Opioid prescribing in the United States before and after the centers for disease control and prevention's 2016 opioid guideline. Ann Intern Med 2018;169(6):367–75.
7. James JR, Scott JM, Klein JW, et al. Mortality after discontinuation of primary care-based chronic opioid therapy for pain: a retrospective cohort study. J Gen Intern Med 2019;34(12):2749–55.
8. Dowell D, Haegerich T, Chou R. No shortcuts to safer opioid prescribing. N Engl J Med 2019;380(24):2285–7.
9. Dowell D, Compton WM, Giroir BP. Patient-centered reduction or discontinuation of long-term opioid analgesics: the HHS guide for clinicians. JAMA 2019;1–3. https://doi.org/10.1001/jama.2019.16409.
10. Dahlhamer J, Lucas J, Zelaya C, et al. Prevalence of chronic pain and high-impact chronic pain among adults - United States, 2016. MMWR Morb Mortal Wkly Rep 2018;67(36):1001–6.
11. Worley SL. New directions in the treatment of chronic pain: national pain strategy will guide prevention, management, and research. P T 2016;41(2):107–14.
12. Chou R, Deyo R, Devine B, et al. The effectiveness and risks of long-term opioid treatment of chronic pain. Evid Rep Technol Assess (Full Rep) 2014;(218):1–219.

13. Krebs EE, Gravely A, Nugent S, et al. Effect of opioid vs nonopioid medications on pain-related function in patients with chronic back pain or hip or knee osteo-arthritis pain: the SPACE randomized clinical trial. JAMA 2018;319(9):872–82.

14. Anastassopoulos KP, Chow W, Tapia CI, et al. Reported side effects, bother, satis-faction, and adherence in patients taking hydrocodone for non-cancer pain. J Opioid Manag 2013;9(2):97–109.

15. Gregorian RS Jr, Gasik A, Kwong WJ, et al. Importance of side effects in opioid treatment: a trade-off analysis with patients and physicians. J Pain 2010;11(11): 1095–108.

16. Thielke SM, Turner JA, Shortreed SM, et al. Do patient-perceived pros and cons of opioids predict sustained higher-dose use? Clin J Pain 2014;30(2):93–101.

17. Yanni LM, McKinney-Ketchum JL, Harrington SB, et al. Preparation, confidence, and attitudes about chronic noncancer pain in graduate medical education. J Grad Med Educ 2010;2(2):260–8.

18. Upshur CC, Luckmann RS, Savageau JA. Primary care provider concerns about management of chronic pain in community clinic populations. J Gen Intern Med 2006;21(6):652–5.

19. Carroll JJ, Colasanti J, Lira MC, et al. HIV physicians and chronic opioid therapy: it's time to raise the bar. AIDS Behav 2019;23(4):1057–61.

20. Jiao JM, So E, Jebakumar J, et al. Chronic pain disorders in HIV primary care: clinical characteristics and association with healthcare utilization. Pain 2016; 157(4):931–7.

21. Bruce RD, Merlin J, Lum PJ, et al. 2017 HIVMA of IDSA clinical practice guideline for the management of chronic pain in patients living with HIV. Clin Infect Dis 2017;65(10):e1–37.

22. Merlin JS, Long D, Becker WC, et al. Brief report: the association of chronic pain and long-term opioid therapy with HIV treatment outcomes. J Acquir Immune Defic Syndr 2018;79(1):77–82.

23. Gardner T, Refshauge K, McAuley J, et al. Patient led goal setting in chronic low back pain-What goals are important to the patient and are they aligned to what we measure? Patient Educ Couns 2015;98(8):1035–8.

24. Schut HA, Stam HJ. Goals in rehabilitation teamwork. Disabil Rehabil 1994;16(4): 223–6.

25. Krebs EE, Lorenz KA, Bair MJ, et al. Development and initial validation of the PEG, a three-item scale assessing pain intensity and interference. J Gen Intern Med 2009;24(6):733–8.

26. Eccleston C, Palermo TM, Williams AC, et al. Psychological therapies for the man-agement of chronic and recurrent pain in children and adolescents. Cochrane Database Syst Rev 2014;(5):CD003968.

27. Williams AC, Eccleston C, Morley S. Psychological therapies for the management of chronic pain (excluding headache) in adults. Cochrane Database Syst Rev 2012;(11):CD007407.

28. Geneen LJ, Moore RA, Clarke C, et al. Physical activity and exercise for chronic pain in adults: an overview of Cochrane Reviews. Cochrane Database Syst Rev 2017;(4):CD011279.

29. Towheed TE, Maxwell L, Judd MG, et al. Acetaminophen for osteoarthritis. Co-chrane Database Syst Rev 2006;1:CD004257.

30. Chou R, Deyo R, Friedly J, et al. Systemic pharmacologic therapies for low back pain: a systematic review for an American College of Physicians clinical practice guideline. Ann Intern Med 2017;166(7):480–92.

31. Enthoven WT, Roelofs PD, Deyo RA, et al. Non-steroidal anti-inflammatory drugs for chronic low back pain. Cochrane Database Syst Rev 2016;2:CD012087.

32. Qaseem A, Wilt TJ, McLean RM, et al. Clinical guidelines committee of the american college of p. noninvasive treatments for acute, subacute, and chronic low back pain: a clinical practice guideline from the American College of Physicians. Ann Intern Med 2017;166(7):514–30.

33. Fanelli A, Ghisi D, Aprile PL, et al. Cardiovascular and cerebrovascular risk with nonsteroidal anti-inflammatory drugs and cyclooxygenase 2 inhibitors: latest evidence and clinical implications. Ther Adv Drug Saf 2017;8(6):173–82.

34. Lanza FL, Chan FK, Quigley EM. Practice Parameters Committee of the American College of G. Guidelines for prevention of NSAID-related ulcer complications. Am J Gastroenterol 2009;104(3):728–38.

35. Scheiman JM, Yeomans ND, Talley NJ, et al. Prevention of ulcers by esomeprazole in at-risk patients using non-selective NSAIDs and COX-2 inhibitors. Am J Gastroenterol 2006;101(4):701–10.

36. Sriperumbuduri S, Hiremath S. The case for cautious consumption: NSAIDs in chronic kidney disease. Curr Opin Nephrol Hypertens 2019;28(2):163–70.

37. Gingras MA, Lieu A, Papillon-Ferland L, et al. Retrospective cohort study of the prevalence of off-label gabapentinoid prescriptions in hospitalized medical patients. J Hosp Med 2019;14:E1–4.

38. Gardea MA, Gatchel RJ. Interdisciplinary treatment of chronic pain. Curr Rev Pain 2000;4(1):18–23.

39. Nicolaidis C. Police officer, deal-maker, or health care provider? Moving to a patient-centered framework for chronic opioid management. Pain Med 2011; 12(6):890–7.

40. Alford DP. Opioid prescribing for chronic pain–achieving the right balance through education. N Engl J Med 2016;374(4):301–3.

41. Chou R, Turner JA, Devine EB, et al. The effectiveness and risks of long-term opioid therapy for chronic pain: a systematic review for a National Institutes of Health Pathways to Prevention Workshop. Ann Intern Med 2015;162(4):276–86.

42. Edelman EJ, Gordon KS, Crothers K, et al. Association of prescribed opioids with increased risk of community-acquired pneumonia among patients with and without HIV. JAMA Intern Med 2019;179(3):297–304.

43. Park TW, Larochelle MR, Saitz R, et al. Associations between prescribed benzodiazepines, overdose death and buprenorphine discontinuation among people receiving buprenorphine. Addiction 2020;115(5):924–32.

44. Dasgupta N, Funk MJ, Proescholdbell S, et al. Cohort study of the impact of high-dose opioid analgesics on overdose mortality. Pain Med 2016;17(1):85–98.

45. Webster LR, Webster RM. Predicting aberrant behaviors in opioid-treated patients: preliminary validation of the Opioid Risk Tool. Pain Med 2005;6(6):432–42.

46. Butler SF, Budman SH, Fernandez K, et al. Validation of a screener and opioid assessment measure for patients with chronic pain. Pain 2004;112(1–2):65–75.

47. Adams LL, Gatchel RJ, Robinson RC, et al. Development of a self-report screening instrument for assessing potential opioid medication misuse in chronic pain patients. J Pain Symptom Manage 2004;27(5):440–59.

48. Butler SF, Budman SH, Fernandez KC, et al. Development and validation of the Current Opioid Misuse Measure. Pain 2007;130(1–2):144–56.

49. Lawrence R, Mogford D, Colvin L. Systematic review to determine which validated measurement tools can be used to assess risk of problematic analgesic use in patients with chronic pain. Br J Anaesth 2017;119(6):1092–109.

50. Starrels JL, Becker WC, Alford DP, et al. Systematic review: treatment agreements and urine drug testing to reduce opioid misuse in patients with chronic pain. Ann Intern Med 2010;152(11):712–20.
51. Rager JB, Schwartz PH. Defending opioid treatment agreements: disclosure, not promises. Hastings Cent Rep 2017;47(3):24–33.
52. Argoff CE, Alford DP, Fudin J, et al. Rational urine drug monitoring in patients receiving opioids for chronic pain: consensus recommendations. Pain Med 2018;19(1):97–117.
53. Haegerich TM, Jones CM, Cote PO, et al. Evidence for state, community and systems-level prevention strategies to address the opioid crisis. Drug Alcohol Depend 2019;204:107563.
54. Hasin DS, O'Brien CP, Auriacombe M, et al. DSM-5 criteria for substance use disorders: recommendations and rationale. Am J Psychiatry 2013;170:834–51.
55. Lin LA, Bohnert ASB, Kerns RD, et al. Impact of the Opioid Safety Initiative on opioid-related prescribing in veterans. Pain 2017;158(5):833–9.
56. Frank JW, Lovejoy TI, Becker WC, et al. Patient outcomes in dose reduction or discontinuation of long-term opioid therapy: a systematic review. Ann Intern Med 2017;167(3):181–91.
57. Berna C, Kulich RJ, Rathmell JP. Tapering long-term opioid therapy in chronic noncancer pain: evidence and recommendations for everyday practice. Mayo Clin Proc 2015;90(6):828–42.
58. Lira MC, Tsui JI, Liebschutz JM, et al. Study protocol for the targeting effective analgesia in clinics for HIV (TEACH) study - a cluster randomized controlled trial and parallel cohort to increase guideline concordant care for long-term opioid therapy among people living with HIV. HIV Res Clin Pract 2019;20(2):48–63.
59. Liebschutz JM, Xuan Z, Shanahan CW, et al. Improving adherence to long-term opioid therapy guidelines to reduce opioid misuse in primary care: a cluster-randomized clinical trial. JAMA Intern Med 2017;177(9):1265–72.
60. Samet JH, Liebschutz J, Cheng DM, et al. Improving Chronic Opioid Therapy Among People Living with HIV: A Clinical RCT. Conference on Retroviruses and Opportunistic Infections. Seattle, Washington. March 4–7, 2019. Abstract #889.
61. Starrels JL, Peyser D, Haughton L, et al. When human immunodeficiency virus (HIV) treatment goals conflict with guideline-based opioid prescribing: A qualitative study of HIV treatment providers. Subst Abus 2016;37(1):148–53.
62. Del Rio C, Tsui JI, Cheng DM, et al. Targeting Effective Analgesia in Clinics for HIV (TEACH): a Randomized Controlled Trial (RCT) to Improve Satisfaction, Confidence, and Trust around Chronic Opioid Therapy in HIV Care. 10th IAS Conference on HIV Science (IAS 2019), Mexico City, July 21–24, 2019. Abstract MOPDB0104.

Lessons Learned from the Response to the Human Immunodeficiency Virus Epidemic that Can Inform Addressing the Opioid Epidemic

Sandra A. Springer, MD[a],*, Carlos del Rio, MD[b]

KEYWORDS

- HIV • Opioid use disorder • Epidemic • Medication treatment of opioid use disorder
- MOUD • HCV • Infectious disease • Stigma

KEY POINTS

- The opioid epidemic is fueling new infectious disease epidemics, including human immunodeficiency virus (HIV), hepatitis C virus, and serious bacterial infections such as infective endocarditis, across the United States among persons who use drugs.
- There are significant parallels with the early years of the HIV epidemic and the current opioid epidemic that are discussed in this article.
- Evidence-based interventions that were implemented in response to the HIV epidemic can also be used to combat the current opioid epidemic and intertwined infectious disease epidemics in the United States.

INTRODUCTION

When people typically hear the word epidemic these days, they envision influenza, Ebola, or now the novel Coronavirus Infectious Disease of 2019 (COVID-19) caused by SARS-CoV-2. According to Wikipedia, an epidemic is "the rapid spread of an infectious disease to a large number of people in a given population within a short period of time." Although OUD is not an infectious disease, its "transmission" mimics infectious diseases and it is directly related to a surge in infectious diseases such as human immunodeficiency virus (HIV), hepatitis C virus (HCV), and serious bacterial infections such as infective endocarditis.

[a] Department of Internal Medicine, Section of Infectious Diseases, AIDS Program, Yale School of Medicine, 135 College Street, Suite 323, New Haven, CT 06510, USA; [b] Department of Medicine, Division of Infectious Diseases, Emory University School of Medicine, 69 Jesse Hill Jr. Dr. Faculty Office Building, Room 201, Atlanta, GA 30303, USA
* Corresponding author.
E-mail address: Sandra.springer@yale.edu

Infect Dis Clin N Am 34 (2020) 637–647
https://doi.org/10.1016/j.idc.2020.06.015
0891-5520/20/© 2020 Elsevier Inc. All rights reserved.
id.theclinics.com

"Access to life-saving interventions must be improved in all settings worldwide" to successfully address epidemics, according to the World Health Organization (WHO).[1] When the HIV epidemic was first recognized in the United States, the response was delayed and stigma and discrimination in society and health care were prominent. In responding to the early HIV epidemic, the US government funded the AIDS (acquired immunodeficiency syndrome) Service Demonstration Grants through the Health Resources and Services Administration (HRSA) in 1986 with $15.3 million dollars targeting the 4 hardest-hit cities: New York, San Francisco, Los Angeles, and Miami. Subsequent funding intended to help communities respond to the epidemic included the azidothymidine (AZT) reimbursement program in 1987, the pediatric AIDS grants in 1988, and the HRSA low-prevalence planning grants in 1989. On August 18, 1990, with bipartisan support, both houses of Congress passed the Ryan White Comprehensive AIDS Resources Emergency (CARE) Act. At that time, more than 150,000 cases and more than 100,000 deaths had been reported. This unprecedented federal funding allowed states and jurisdictions to integrate efforts necessary to provide access to care and support and, beginning in 1996, to life-saving antiretroviral therapy (ART) for persons living with HIV (PLWH). However, despite the advances in prevention and care that have reduced mortality from HIV/AIDS by more than 80% since it peaked in 1995 and have decreased new infections by 8% since 2010, there are still approximately 38,500 people newly infected each year, and new HIV outbreaks are now occurring across the country among persons who use drugs (PWUD). There seems to be a collective amnesia about this earlier HIV epidemic and the well-documented relationship between heroin use and injection drug use (IDU) along with condomless sexual intercourse that fueled the HIV epidemic then among PWUD. However, the successful skills and evidence-based tools in identifying, treating, and preventing HIV at this time, including what is needed by the WHO to combat an epidemic, access to life-saving medication treatments, is not being used for persons living with OUD. As this article describes, the lessons learned from the HIV epidemic need to be used to overcome this current opioid epidemic and intertwined HIV, HCV, as well as invasive bacterial and fungal infectious disease epidemics in this country.

BACKGROUND
Current State of the Problem

According to the National Institute of Drug Abuse (NIDA), there are currently more than 2.1 million persons with OUD in this country, with only approximately 20% receiving treatment. In October 2017, the President of the United States declared the opioid epidemic a national public health emergency. This epidemic has been manifested by a dramatic increase in the nonmedical use and abuse of prescription opioids, an increase in heroin use,[2] a large number of opioid overdose deaths,[3] and a tripling of emergency department visits because of opioid overdose.[4] In 2017, more than 47,600 Americans died of opioid overdoses, which was the leading cause of accidental death in the United States, surpassing motor vehicle accidents and gun deaths.[5] According to the Centers for Disease Control and Prevention (CDC), it is estimated that every day 130 individuals die of overdosing on opioids.[6,7] In particular the concern is the increase of illicitly manufactured fentanyl used in isolation or with other drugs, such as the stimulants methamphetamine and cocaine, that are causing an alarming number of deaths nationally.[8,9] Although the latest data released recently have shown a slight decrease of overall national overdose deaths (4.6%) from 2017 to 2018, there are significant variations across the states, with some having marked increases in deaths caused by opioid overdoses and others reporting slight decreases in deaths caused by opioid overdoses.[7] In particular, a more granular level of evaluation by the CDC has shown a decrease in prescription opioid overdoses, whereas there was a marked increase in deaths caused by illicitly manufactured fentanyl overdoses, especially in people who used multiple illicit opioids and nonopioids. Illicitly manufactured fentanyl was involved in approximately two-thirds of opioid deaths during January to June 2018, and during this time more than 60% of all opioid deaths nationally co-occurred with at least 1 common nonopioid drug such as methamphetamine, cocaine, or benzodiazapines.[7]

In addition to the direct deaths caused by opioids and other drugs occurring at unprecedented levels, the opioid epidemic has resulted in an increase in infections among PWUD,[10–15] magnifying the morbidity and mortality associated with illicit opioid and other substance use. Such infections that are increasing related to illicit opioid and other drug use include HCV; hepatitis B virus; HIV; and invasive bacterial and fungal infections, including *Staphylococcus aureus* bacteremia, endocarditis, skin and soft tissue infections, and bone and joint infections.[10,13,16–18] Fentanyl or heroin combined with stimulants such as cocaine and methamphetamine have led to new HIV outbreaks among PWUD throughout the country[13–15] as well as increased overdose deaths.[19] Further, opioid addiction impedes patients from staying adherent to effective treatments when they are provided and thus leads to readmissions as well as death caused by persistent or untreated infections.

This population with co-occurring IDU-related infections represents the most severely ill patients with OUD, and an important opportunity to intervene, both to improve patients' outcomes and to reduce the public health risk of infectious disease transmission. Further, OUD affects everyone: people from urban, suburban, and rural communities alike; persons at all income levels; all racial and ethnic minorities; all age groups, with younger persons being affected substantially; and persons with mental illness.[20] Infectious disease physicians as well as other physicians and nonphysician clinicians are at the forefront of these coalescing epidemics. Infectious disease clinicians are most likely to have learned lessons from the original HIV epidemic to help to defeat the opioid epidemic.

The Human Immunodeficiency Virus Epidemic in 1980s to 1990s in the United States

In the early 1980s and 1990s, the United States was experiencing one of the worst epidemics in the country's history, the HIV epidemic. Initially identified among young men who had sex with men, it was quickly recognized among heterosexual men and women, children, and persons who injected or used drugs.[21] The early HIV epidemic associated with IDU was related to injection of heroin and cocaine and affected persons predominantly living in urban centers and afflicting mainly African American and Hispanic men and women.[22,23] In the beginning of the epidemic, even after HIV was identified as the cause of AIDS, medication development was slow, and the medications were expensive and difficult to access. It was not until the mid-1990s that effective combination ART was identified with the discovery of the class of ART called protease inhibitors, which, when used in combination with nucleoside reverse transcriptase inhibitors, reduced deaths among PLWH. Issues originally confronting PLWH in terms of access to these lifesaving ART regimens included lack of insurance and/or lack of access to the expensive medications; high levels of stigma,[24] not only in the community but among providers, including infectious disease physicians who were at the forefront of the epidemic; and, in general, a lack of provider workforce or willingness to treat PLWH.[25]

More persons have now died of the opioid epidemic than have died at the height of the AIDS epidemic in the United States.[26] The current opioid epidemic began in the late 1990s, associated with addiction to prescription opioids prescribed by clinicians for treatment of pain disorders. In 2015, a new HIV and HCV outbreak occurred in Scott County, Indiana, specifically linked with prescription opioid misuse in the United States.[13] This HIV and HCV epidemic was identified through the CDC to be linked directly to both sharing contaminated IDU works when injecting oxymorphone (Opana) as well as through condomless sexual intercourse.[27]

Over time, there was a change from addiction to prescription opioids to a new heroin epidemic across the country, which was predominantly found to involve the rapidly available and less expensive black tar heroin coming from Mexico,[28] which in turn led to another spike in overdose deaths and associated with more HCV and HIV outbreaks nationally. It is important to remember that the early HIV epidemic was associated with white heroin from Asia, which had low supply levels in the United States back then and was predominantly affecting urban African Americans.[28] Very little public outcry was heard and, in response, there was a war on drugs that led to the country's mass incarceration of predominantly PWUD, who were predominantly young African American men. In comparison, the current opioid epidemic is affecting urban and rural communities among mainly young white men and women. Later, the opioid epidemic worsened again with the availability of the less expensive illicitly manufactured fentanyl, and this epidemic has been plaguing the country in isolation as well as now more routinely associated with an increasing stimulant epidemic involving widespread use of methamphetamine, which is causing even more overdose deaths and more infectious disease outbreaks without any evidence of abating.[9,29] The reason the United States did not have a rapidly expanding opioid epidemic in the 1970s and 1980s was predominantly that there was a lack of widespread opioid supply, but, with the rapidly expanding prescription opioid epidemic, the supply increased dramatically in the late 1990s, leading to rapid opioid addiction by persons affected by OUD that was easily fulfilled by the less expensive and easily available black tar heroin that was supplied through Mexico and now the illicitly manufactured fentanyl.[28,30]

Although it is not surprising, it is still heart breaking for clinicians who cared then and care now for people with HIV (PWH) to see more HIV outbreaks occurring in the United States among PWUD related to these newer opioid epidemics over the past 10 years given that it was known then that sharing contaminated IDU equipment and condomless sexual intercourse drove the HIV epidemic in this country and globally.[22,23,31,32] What is surprising is that, unlike the early HIV epidemic, where there were very few medications to treat HIV early on, for more than 50 years there have been effective medications to treat OUD, including methadone, followed later by buprenorphine, and then extended-release naltrexone. All of these US Food and Drug Administration (FDA)–approved medications have extensive evidence to show that they reduce opioid use, craving, overdose, and HIV and HCV transmission.[33] What is clear is that persons with OUD are not receiving these medications. Further, as was identified at the height of the AIDS epidemic in the United States, harm reduction services such as clean needle syringe exchange programs markedly reduced HIV transmission in PWUD,[34,35] but few programs exist in the United States and, as yet, federal dollars are not provided to purchase syringes. In February 2019, the President of the United States called for a plan to end HIV in the United States, with specific goals to reduce new HIV infections by 75% by 2025 and by 90% by 2030.[36] If these goals are to be achieved, effectively addressing the opioid epidemic is urgently needed: an all-hands-on-deck approach is required.

What Helped in the Human Immunodeficiency Virus Epidemic?

There were several things that happened to effectively begin to address the HIV epidemic early on, but the most impactful event was when Congress passed CARE Act on August 18, 1990.[37] This program allowed specific funding by the federal government to cities, counties, states, and local community-based programs to offer a comprehensive system of HIV primary care, case-management support services, housing assistance, substance use disorder (SUD) treatment, psychosocial behavioral health, wraparound services, and ART.[38]

The CARE Act continues to be critically important in supporting services for the uninsured and underinsured, especially in non-Medicaid expansion states.[37] Importantly, the CARE Act also demanded that acceptance of funding by state programs required that they in turn had to report success metrics to and abide by the provision of ART and the wraparound services. This funding mechanism was instrumental in increasing the workforce because funded programs had to train and hire health care providers to treat PWH. The federal government also funded the AIDS Training and Education Centers (AETCs) beginning in 1987 with the mission of providing health care providers with education on HIV and comorbidities. The AETCs in 1997 became part of the CARE Act. As a result of addressing HIV from diagnosis to viral suppression, the HIV care continuum has been defined with specific outcomes including diagnosis of HIV; linkage to care; ART prescription; ART retention; and, most importantly and the goal of ART treatment, HIV viral suppression.[39] In particular, it is well known that HIV viral suppression not only reduces morbidity and mortality related to HIV-related and non–HIV-related diseases but also reduces HIV transmission to the uninfected.[40] Thus, overall, this evaluation process of the metrics used in the continuum of care provided usable data that supported PWH and improved individual and public health, and essentially upended the increasing HIV epidemic in this country. Programs that received Ryan White funding improved viral suppression rates among PWH from 69.5% to 85.9% from 2010 to 2017 and predominantly among racial/ethnic minorities,[41] and there was a reduction in new HIV infections of 8% from 2010 to 2018, from 41,000 to 37,832.[42] This reduction was caused not only by widespread HIV care through CARE Act–funded programs but also through advances in science, including preexposure prophylaxis to persons at risk for acquiring HIV,[43] the Patient Protection and Affordable Care Act (ACA), the AIDS Drug Assistance Program, and significant research funded by the National Institutes of Health (NIH) and CDC. The requirements of providing services to treat HIV and providing funding for medications to treat HIV with wraparound services such as mental health treatment and SUD treatment have thus led to a reduction in morbidity and mortality from HIV as well as a reduction in new HIV infections in the United States.

In addition to these actions, as well as the CDC's recommendations for universal HIV screening and linkage to care in the United States,[44] specific efforts by The Substance Abuse and Mental Health Services Administration and activism in the community to help programs reduce, but not eliminate, stigma in the general community and among the medical community also helped increase the identification of PWH and provide them immediate care in nonstigmatized environments.[45,46] Stigma was also reduced in this population for explicitly understanding and colocating HIV care along with mental health, SUD care, and case-management services. Further, the harm reduction efforts in particular were highly helpful in transmission of HIV among PWUD through the support of syringe service programs nationally and globally. Education of medical students and other health care students also helped expand HIV care and reduce stigma.[47]

Similarities of the Human Immunodeficiency Virus Epidemic to the Opioid Epidemic

The opioid epidemic parallels the early HIV epidemic in the United States, and clinicians have the tools to combat the epidemic and have had them for some time, but the issue is that they are not being used. Just like HIV disease, persons affected by SUDs and OUD specifically experience high levels of stigma such that it impedes their ability to ask for and receive care. The negative stigma from clinicians is as severe as it was from providers at the height of the AIDS epidemic and, in part, is caused by inadequate training of the clinical workforce on OUD being seen as a character flaw rather than a medical disorder. However, many clinicians view OUD and other SUDs as bad choices by the individual rather than what it is: a medical disorder that is responsive to effective evidence-based treatment.

Further, routine OUD screening and SUD screening in general is not offered universally, much like early in the HIV epidemic.[48] However, there are available screening tools for evaluation of OUD, including the Rapid Opioid dependency Screen (RODS)[49] and others.[50,51] Similar to universal HIV screening services that helped identify and link PLWH to treatment providers, universal OUD screening could be offered to all persons, and those with positive OUD screens could be linked to medication treatment of OUD (MOUD).

However, few persons with OUD are linked to OUD or SUD treatment and, if they are, few providers are approved to prescribe evidence-based FDA-approved MOUD.[33] The 3 FDA-approved MOUDs (methadone, buprenorphine, and extended-release naltrexone [XR-NTX]) are successful in treating OUD through reduction in opioid craving, relapse, and overdose, and they reduce transmission of HIV and HCV[33,52]; buprenorphine and XR-NTX also improve HIV viral suppression in PLWH,[53–55] the gold standard of care in treatment of HIV, which is associated with reduced mortality and reduced transmission[40,54,55] (known as undetectable = untransmittable). In the early years of the HIV epidemic, there was no effective ART, whereas, in the OUD epidemic, there is effective therapy but few are accessing it. The reasons include lack of insurance provisions in non-Medicaid expansion states for SUD treatment; prior authorization requirements to prescribe buprenorphine, or making it mandatory to provide behavioral treatment in order to receive MOUD; Drug Addiction Treatment Act (DATA) 2000 X-waiver mandatory training, which has been identified as burdensome and inadequate as well as placing limitations on the number of persons who can be prescribed buprenorphine; lack of same-day billing for an OUD treatment and other potential associated medical conditions that might require patients to come back another time and expose them to ongoing opioid use and thus increased risk of overdose death or acquisition of infectious diseases; inadequate training of medical professionals and lack of providers to take on treatment; lack of harm reduction expansion services or of federal funding for syringes; and stigma in the general community and across the medical community.[48,56,57]

DISCUSSION
What Can Be Done?

The scrutiny of the parallel of the HIV and the OUD epidemics is helpful because it identifies similar barriers to treatment and how to quell the coalescing substance use and infectious disease epidemics. A recent National Academy of Sciences, Engineering, and Medicine (NASEM) committee has released recommendations identifying these barriers after conducting interviews of programs across the country that were integrating infectious disease and OUD prevention and treatment services.[48,58] In addition, the Infectious Disease Society of America (IDSA) and HIV Medicine Association (HIVMA) working groups also identified similar barriers and made recommendations to directly end both the opioid and associated HIV and other infectious disease epidemics.[59] Such parallels of the opioid epidemic to the early HIV epidemic have led agencies and experts with expertise in HIV and the OUD to call for specific known recommendations to end not only the opioid epidemic but also new illicit substance epidemics, as well as to prevent new HIV and other infectious disease epidemics from occurring in this country, as identified earlier.

In order to end the opioid epidemic, history must be remembered and the lessons learned in combatting the HIV epidemic then applied to combatting the opioid epidemic now. All hands on deck are needed, and now!

SUMMARY

In order to effectively address the opioid epidemic, several important actions are urgently needed:

1. Increasing access to MOUD (buprenorphine, methadone, and extended-release naltrexone) is urgently needed to treat persons with OUD, which means that federal and local government agencies should provide funding to access these medications through Medicaid or local state government , similar to how the CARE Act provided funding for ART for PLWH.
2. Expanding training and education of all health care professionals from students through practicing providers in all disciplines (physicians of all disciplines, nurses, physician assistants, dentist, pharmacists, midwives) regarding how to screen, diagnose, and treat OUD and other SUDs is needed.
3. Removal of federal and local barriers to accessing treatment of OUD, including removal of the DATA 2000 X-waiver mandatory training to provide buprenorphine and removal of limitations of numbers of persons with OUD who can be treated by a provider, are needed to combat the opioid epidemic.
4. Removal of prior authorizations that are burdensome to doctors and also impede the ability to provide in-the-moment appropriate life-saving medication treatment of OUD when a patient requests it is needed.
5. Successful directed stigma reduction regarding persons living with OUDs and substance use in general is required to combat the opioid epidemic, and this involves all persons, including providers, administrators, the community, the media, and patients.
6. Accessible widespread harm reduction services are needed to combat the dueling opioid and HIV epidemics, especially in light of the polysubstance epidemics that include an increase in methamphetamine use, that does not have effective medications to treat it. Thus, services must expand to provide clean syringes, fentanyl testing, and naloxone distribution. Further, federal dollars should be released to states to fund provision of the syringes, fentanyl test strips, and naloxone, along with the staff to provide them.

DISCLOSURE

S.A. Springer has provided scientific consulting to Alkermes Inc. and received NIH funding for research grants. C. del Rio has received research grants from NIH. This research was funded by the National Institute on Drug Abuse (K02 DA032322 for Springer's career development). The funders were not involved in the research design, analysis, or interpretation of the data, or the decision to publish the article. The authors report no conflicts of interest. The authors alone are responsible for the content and writing of this article.

REFERENCES

1. World Health Organization. Managing epidemics: Key Facts about Major Deadly Diseases. 2018.
2. Han B, Compton WM, Jones CM, et al. Nonmedical prescription opioid use and use disorders among adults aged 18 through 64 years in the United States, 2003-2013. JAMA 2015;314:1468–78.
3. Botticelli M. America's Addiction to Opioids: Heroin and Prescription Drug Abuse. 2014. Available at: http://www.drugcaucus.senate.gov/sites/default/files/Botticelli%20Testimony.pdf.
4. Substance Abuse and Mental Health Services Administration. Drug Abuse Warning Network, 2011: National Estimates of Drug-Related Emergency Department Visits. In: Substance Abuse and Mental Health Services Administration, editor. Washington, DC, 2013. Available at: http://www.samhsa.gov/data/2k13/DAWN2k11ED/DAWN2k11ED.htm#5.2.
5. Rudd RA, Seth P, David F, et al. Increases in drug and opioid-involved overdose deaths - United States, 2010-2015. MMWR Morb Mortal Wkly Rep 2016;65:1445–52.
6. National Institute of Drug Abuse. Over Dose Rates. September 2017. 2017. Available at: https://www.drugabuse.gov/related-topics/trends-statistics/overdose-death-rates. Accessed January 3, 2019.
7. Gladden RM, O'Donnell J, Mattson CL, et al. Changes in Opioid-Involved Overdose Deaths by Opioid Type and Presence of Benzodiazepines, Cocaine, and Methamphetamine - 25 States, July-December 2017 to January-June 2018. MMWR Morb Mortal Wkly Rep 2019;68:737–44.
8. Zoorob M. Fentanyl shock: The changing geography of overdose in the United States. Int J Drug Policy 2019;70:40–6.
9. Kariisa M, Scholl L, Wilson N, et al. Drug overdose deaths involving cocaine and psychostimulants with abuse potential - United States, 2003-2017. MMWR Morb Mortal Wkly Rep 2019;68:388–95.
10. Ronan MV, Herzig SJ. Hospitalizations related to opioid abuse/dependence and associated serious infections increased sharply, 2002-12. Health Aff (Millwood) 2016;35:832–7.
11. Fleischauer AT, Ruhl L, Rhea S, et al. Hospitalizations for endocarditis and associated health care costs among persons with diagnosed drug dependence - North Carolina, 2010-2015. MMWR Morb Mortal Wkly Rep 2017;66:569–73.
12. Jackson KA, Bohm MK, Brooks JT, et al. Invasive methicillin-resistant staphylococcus aureus infections among persons who inject drugs - six sites, 2005-2016. MMWR Morb Mortal Wkly Rep 2018;67:625–8.
13. Conrad C, Bradley HM, Broz D, et al. Community Outbreak of HIV infection linked to injection drug use of oxymorphone–Indiana, 2015. MMWR Morb Mortal Wkly Rep 2015;64:443–4.
14. Cranston K, Alpren C, John B, et al. Notes from the Field: HIV Diagnoses Among Persons Who Inject Drugs - Northeastern Massachusetts, 2015-2018. MMWR Morb Mortal Wkly Rep 2019;68:253–4.
15. Golden MR, Lechtenberg R, Glick SN, et al. Outbreak of Human Immunodeficiency Virus Infection Among Heterosexual Persons Who Are Living Homeless

and Inject Drugs - Seattle, Washington, 2018. MMWR Morb Mortal Wkly Rep 2019;68:344–9.

16. Zibbell JE, Asher AK, Patel RC, et al. Increases in acute hepatitis C virus infection related to a growing opioid epidemic and associated injection drug use, United States, 2004 to 2014. Am J Public Health 2018;108:175–81.

17. Schranz AJ, Fleischauer A, Chu VH, et al. Trends in drug use-associated infective endocarditis and heart valve surgery, 2007 to 2017: a study of statewide discharge data. Ann Intern Med 2018;170(1):31–40.

18. Wurcel AG, Anderson JE, Chui KK, et al. Increasing infectious endocarditis admissions among young people who inject drugs. Open Forum Infect Dis 2016; 3:ofw157.

19. Ruhm C. Nonopioid overdose death rates rose almost as fast as those involving opioids, 1999–2016. Health Aff 2019;38:1216–24.

20. Centers for Disease Control (CDC). Risk Factors for Prescription Painkiller Abuse and Overdose. 2015.

21. Curran JW, Jaffe HW, Centers for Disease C, Prevention. AIDS: the early years and CDC's response. MMWR Suppl 2011;60:64–9.

22. Des Jarlais DC, Kerr T, Carrieri P, et al. HIV infection among persons who inject drugs: ending old epidemics and addressing new outbreaks. AIDS 2016;30: 815–26.

23. Des Jarlais DC, Carrieri P. HIV infection among persons who inject drugs: ending old epidemics and addressing new outbreaks: authors' reply. AIDS 2016;30: 1858–9.

24. Mahajan AP, Sayles JN, Patel VA, et al. Stigma in the HIV/AIDS epidemic: a review of the literature and recommendations for the way forward. AIDS 2008;22(Suppl 2):S67–79.

25. Fox DM. AIDS and the American Health Polity: the history and prospects of a crisis of authority. Millbank Q 2005;83(4):1–26.

26. DeWeerdt S. Tracing the US opioid crisis to its roots. Nature 2019;573:S10–2.

27. Peters PJ, Pontones P, Hoover KW, et al. HIV infection linked to injection use of oxymorphone in Indiana, 2014-2015. N Engl J Med 2016;375:229–39.

28. Quinones S. Dreamland. 1st edition. New York: Bloomsbury Press; 2015.

29. Rudd RA, Paulozzi LJ, Bauer MJ, et al. Increases in heroin overdose deaths - 28 States, 2010 to 2012. MMWR Morb Mortal Wkly Rep 2014;63:849–54.

30. Ciccarone D. The triple wave epidemic: Supply and demand drivers of the US opioid overdose crisis. Int J Drug Policy 2019;71:183–8.

31. Des Jarlais DC, Friedman SR, Novick DM, et al. HIV-1 infection among intravenous drug users in Manhattan, New York City, from 1977 through 1987. JAMA 1989;261:1008–12.

32. Des Jarlais DC, Feelemyer JP, Modi SN, et al. Are females who inject drugs at higher risk for HIV infection than males who inject drugs: an international systematic review of high seroprevalence areas. Drug Alcohol Depend 2012;124: 95–107.

33. SAMHSA. Tip 63: medications for opioid use disorder-executive summary. Washington, DC: Department of Health and Human Services; 2018.

34. Beg M, Strathdee SA, Kazatchkine M. State of the art science addressing injecting drug use, HIV and harm reduction. Int J Drug Policy 2015;26(Suppl 1):S1–4.

35. Abdul-Quader AS, Feelemyer J, Modi S, et al. Effectiveness of structural-level needle/syringe programs to reduce HCV and HIV infection among people who inject drugs: a systematic review. AIDS Behav 2013;17(9):2878–92.

36. HRSA. What is 'Ending the HIV Epidemic: A Plan for America'? 2019. Available at: https://www.hiv.gov/federal-response/ending-the-hiv-epidemic/overview.

37. Congress US. Ryan White HIV/AIDS Program Legislation. 1990. Available at: https://hab.hrsa.gov/about-ryan-white-hivaids-program/ryan-white-hivaids-program-legislation.

38. Kay ES, Batey DS, Mugavero MJ. The ryan white HIV/AIDS program: supplementary service provision post-affordable care act. AIDS Patient Care STDS 2018;32: 265–71.

39. Colasanti J, Kelly J, Pennisi E, et al. Continuous Retention and Viral Suppression Provide Further Insights Into the HIV Care Continuum Compared to the Cross-sectional HIV Care Cascade. Clin Infect Dis 2016;62:648–54.

40. Cohen MS, Chen YQ, McCauley M, et al. Prevention of HIV-1 infection with early antiretroviral therapy. N Engl J Med 2011;365:493–505.

41. Health Resources and Services Administration (HRSA). Ryan White HIV/AIDS program annual client-level data report 2017. In: Administration HRaS, editor. Washington, DC: Health Resources and Services Administration (HRSA); 2018.

42. Centers for Disease Control and Prevention (CDC). Diagnoses of HIV infection in the United States and dependent areas, 2018. Atlanta (GA): (CDC); 2018.

43. Centers for Disease Control and Prevention (CDC). Preexposure Prophylaxis for the prevention of HIV infection in the United States-2014: a Clinical Practice Guideline. Bethesda (MD): DHHS) United States Department of Health and Human Services (DHHS); 2014.

44. Centers for Disease Control and Prevention. Revised recommendations for HIv testing of adults, adolescents, and pregnant women in health-care settings. MMWR Morb Mortal Wkly Rep 2006;55:1–17.

45. Stangl AL, Lloyd JK, Brady LM, et al. A systematic review of interventions to reduce HIV-related stigma and discrimination from 2002 to 2013: how far have we come? J Int AIDS Soc 2013;16:18734.

46. Gruskin S, Tarantola D. Universal Access to HIV prevention, treatment and care: assessing the inclusion of human rights in international and national strategic plans. AIDS 2008;22(Suppl 2):S123–32.

47. Nyblade L, Stangl A, Weiss E, et al. Combating HIV stigma in health care settings: what works? J Int AIDS Soc 2009;12:15.

48. National Academies of Sciences, Engineering, and Medicine. Opportunities to improve opioid use disorder and infectious disease services: Integrating responses to a dual epidemic. In: The National Academies of Science, Engineering, and Medicine, editor. Washington, DC: The National Academies Press; 2020. Available at: http://nationalacademies.org/hmd/Activities/PublicHealth/ExaminationoftheIntegrationofOpioidandInfectiousDiseasePreventionEffortsin SelectPrograms.aspx.

49. Wickersham JA, Azar MM, Cannon CM, et al. Validation of a brief measure of opioid dependence: the rapid opioid dependence screen (RODS). J Correct Health Care 2015;21:12–26.

50. Seval N, Eaton E, Springer SA. Beyond antibiotics: a practical guide for the infectious disease physician to treat opioid use disorder in the setting of associated infectious diseases. Open Forum Infect Dis 2020;7:ofz539.

51. Seval N, Eaton E, Springer SA. Inpatient Opioid Use Disorder (OUD) treatment for the infectious disease physician. In: Norton B, editor. The opioid epidemic and infectious diseases. 1st edition. New York: Elsevier Inc.; 2020.

52. Gowing L, Farrell MF, Bornemann R, et al. Oral substitution treatment of injecting opioid users for prevention of HIV infection. Cochrane Database Syst Rev 2011;(8):CD004145.
53. Springer SA, Chen S, Altice FL. Improved HIV and substance abuse treatment outcomes for released HIV-infected prisoners: the impact of buprenorphine treatment. J Urban Health 2010;87:592–602.
54. Springer SA, Di Paola A, Azar MM, et al. Extended-release naltrexone improves viral suppression among incarcerated persons living with HIV with opioid use disorders transitioning to the community: results of a double-blind, placebo-controlled randomized trial. J Acquir Immune Defic Syndr 2018;78:43–53.
55. Springer SA, Qiu J, Saber-Tehrani AS, et al. Retention on buprenorphine is associated with high levels of maximal viral suppression among HIV-infected opioid dependent released prisoners. PLoS One 2012;7:e38335.
56. Springer SA, Korthuis PT, Del Rio C. Integrating treatment at the intersection of opioid use disorder and infectious disease epidemics in medical settings: a call for action after a national academies of sciences, engineering, and medicine workshop. Ann Intern Med 2018;169:335–6.
57. National Academies of Sciences, Engineering, and Medicine. Integrating responses at the Intersection of Opioid Use Disorder and Infectious Disease Epidemics: Proceedings of a Workshop. In: National Academies of Sciences, Engineering, and Medicine, editor. Washington, DC: National Academies of Sciences, Engineering, and Medicine; 2018. Available at: http://www.nationalacademies.org/hmd/Reports/2018/integrating-responses-at-the-intersection-of-opioid-use-disorder-and-infectious-disease-epidemics-proceedings.aspx.
58. Springer SA, Merluzzi AP, Del Rio C. Integrating Responses to the Opioid Use Disorder and Infectious Disease Epidemics: A Report From the National Academies of Sciences, Engineering, and Medicine. JAMA 2020. Available at: https://www.ncbi.nlm.nih.gov/pubmed/32159771.
59. Reducing the Infectious Consequences of Substance Use Disorders: An Urgent Call to Action from the Infectious Disease Society of America (IDSA) and HIV Medicine Association (HIVMA). Journal Of Infectious Disease. September 2020. In Press.

Moving?

Make sure your subscription moves with you!

To notify us of your new address, find your **Clinics Account Number** (located on your mailing label above your name), and contact customer service at:

Email: journalscustomerservice-usa@elsevier.com

800-654-2452 (subscribers in the U.S. & Canada)
314-447-8871 (subscribers outside of the U.S. & Canada)

Fax number: 314-447-8029

Elsevier Health Sciences Division
Subscription Customer Service
3251 Riverport Lane
Maryland Heights, MO 63043

*To ensure uninterrupted delivery of your subscription, please notify us at least 4 weeks in advance of move.

ELSEVIER